BRASSICA GERMPLASM - CHARACTERIZATION, BREEDING AND UTILIZATION

Edited by **Mohamed Ahmed El-Esawi**

Brassica Germplasm - Characterization, Breeding and Utilization
http://dx.doi.org/10.5772/intechopen.71706
Edited by Mohamed Ahmed El-Esawi

Contributors

Haq Nawaz, Muhammad Aslam Shad, Saima Muzaffar, Vagner Arnaut De Toledo, Emerson Dechechi Chambó, Simone Camargo, Maria Claudia Ruvolo-Takasusuki, Ludimilla Ronqui, Pedro Santos, Claudio Silva Júnior, Carlos A Carvalho, Regina Garcia, Muhammad Imran, Giuseppina Lima, Santino Seabra Junior, Cristine Vanz Borges, Franciely Da Silva Ponce, Namiko Nishida, Ryo Fujimoto, Ayasha Akter, Satoko Takada, Etsuko Itabashi, Kenji Osabe, Daniel John Shea, Vladimir Meglič, Barbara Pipan, Ana-Alexandra Sorescu, Alexandrina Nuta, Rodica-Mariana Ion, Mohamed A. El-Esawi

First published in London, United Kingdom, 2018 by IntechOpen
IntechOpen is the global imprint of INTECHOPEN LIMITED, registered in England and Wales, registration number: 11086078, The Shard, 25th floor, 32 London Bridge Street
London, SE19SG – United Kingdom
Printed in Croatia

British Library Cataloguing-in-Publication Data
A catalogue record for this book is available from the British Library

Additional hard copies can be obtained from orders@intechopen.com

Brassica Germplasm - Characterization, Breeding and Utilization, Edited by Mohamed Ahmed El-Esawi
p. cm.
Print ISBN 978-1-78984-241-8
Online ISBN 978-1-78984-242-5

For EU product safety concerns:
IN TECH d.o.o., Prolaz Marije Krucifikse Kozulić 3, 51000 Rijeka, Croatia,
info@intechopen.com or visit our website at intechopen.com.

Meet the editor

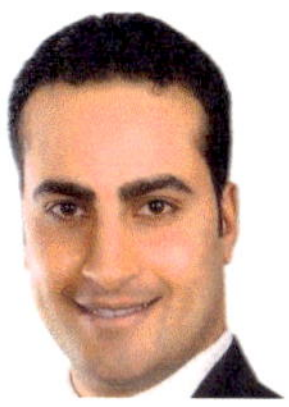

Dr. Mohamed Ahmed El-Esawi is currently a visiting research fellow at the University of Cambridge in the United Kingdom, and an associate professor of Molecular Genetics at the Botany Department of Tanta University in Egypt. Dr. El-Esawi received his BSc and MSc degrees from Tanta University, and his PhD degree in Plant Genetics and Molecular Biology from Dublin Institute of Technology in Ireland. Afterwards, Dr. El-Esawi joined The University of Warwick in the UK, University of Sorbonne (Paris VI) in France, and University of Leuven (KU Leuven) in Belgium as a visiting research fellow. His research focuses on plant genetics, genomics, molecular biology, molecular physiology, developmental biology, plant-microbe interaction and bioinformatics. He has authored several international journal articles and book chapters and participated in more than 60 conferences and workshops worldwide. Dr. El-Esawi is currently involved in several research projects on biological sciences.

Contents

Preface

The genus *Brassica* L. of the family Brassicaceae has a vital role in agriculture and human health. The genus comprises of several species, including major oilseed and vegetable crops with promising agronomic traits. *Brassica* species are vital resources of vegetable oil, vegetables and condiments. *Brassica napus, B. rapa, B. juncea* and *B. carinata* provide approximately 12% of the vegetable oil supply worldwide. The oil is utilized for human consumption or as a biofuel or renewable resource in the petrochemical industry. Brassicaceae contains glucosinolates that are broken down to isothiocyanates and these are known to mitigate tumour development and prevent a range of heart diseases and human cancers. The plants comprising high amounts of glucosinolate may be further utilized as a potential genetic source for breeding. *Brassica* secondary products have antibacterial, antioxidant and antiviral effects. Characterization of *Brassica* is important for providing information on domestication, propagation and breeding programs, as well as conservation of plant genetic resources.

This book highlights the current knowledge of the genus *Brassica* L. in order to understand its biology, diversity, conservation and breeding, as well as to develop disease-resistant and more productive crops. Breeding technologies and resistance to abiotic stresses in *Brassica* species are also discussed. This book will be of interest to many readers, researchers and scientists, who will find this information useful for the advancement of their research towards a better understanding of *Brassica* breeding programs.

The book includes ten chapters, which provide up-to-date knowledge on *Brassica* genetic resources. The titles of the ten chapters are as follows: (1) Characterization and Breeding of *Brassica* Germplasm, (2) Phytochemical Composition and Antioxidant Potential of *Brassica*, (3) Spatial and Temporal Assessment of *Brassica napus* L. Maintaining Genetic Diversity and Gene Flow Potential: An Empirical Evaluation, (4) Glucosinolates in Brassicas, (5) Vegetable *Brassica* Breeding, (6) Pale-Green Kohlrabi, a Versatile *Brassica* Vegetable, (7) Agronomic Factors Influencing *Brassica* Productivity and Phytochemical Quality, (8) Genetic and Epigenetic Regulation of Vernalization in Brassicaceae, (9) Benefits of Entomophile Pollination in Crops of *Brassica napus* and Aspects of Plant Floral Biology, and (10) Economic Insect Pests of *Brassica*.

The book editor would like to thank Ms. Marijana Francetic, Publishing Process Manager, for her wholehearted cooperation in the publication of this book.

Mohamed Ahmed El-Esawi, PhD
Botany Department
Faculty of Science
Tanta University, Egypt

Sainsbury Laboratory
University of Cambridge
Cambridge, United Kingdom

Chapter 1

Introductory Chapter: Characterization and Breeding of *Brassica* Germplasm

Mohamed A. El-Esawi

Additional information is available at the end of the chapter

http://dx.doi.org/10.5772/intechopen.80457

1. Introduction

The genus *Brassica* L. belonging to the family Brassicaceae has a vital role in agriculture and populations health [1]. It comprises several species, including major oilseed and vegetable crops of promising agronomic traits [2–5]. *Brassica* species are vital resources of vegetable oil, vegetables, and condiments [6]. *Brassica napus*, *B. rapa*, *B. juncea*, and *B. carinata* provide approximately 12% of the vegetable oil supply worldwide [3, 7]. The oil is utilized for human consumption or as a biofuel or renewable resource in the petrochemical industry. *B. oleracea* comprises a large storage capacity for nutrients and provides a large range of unique cole and cabbage crops used for human consumption [1, 3]. The seed of *Brassica nigra* is used as a condiment mustard. Furthermore, *Brassica* species are vital sources of potassium; dietary fiber; vitamins A, C, and E; phenolics; and other health-enhancing factors [3, 6, 8]. Brassicaceae contains glucosinolates which are broken down to isothiocyanates known to mitigate tumor development and resist a range of heart diseases and human cancers [2, 3, 9]. The plants comprising high amount of glucosinolate may be further utilized as a potential genetic source for breeding [10]. *Brassica* vegetables inhibit major diseases such as Alzheimer's, and some of the functional declines associated with aging [3, 9].

Brassica secondary products have antibacterial, antioxidant, and antiviral effects as well as inducing the immune system and regulating steroid metabolism [2, 3, 9]. Various fungal, bacterial, viral, and insect and pest pathogens, including *Plasmodiophora brassicae* (clubroot), *Peronospora parasitica* (downy mildew), *Ophiosphaerella korrae* (ring spot), *Leptosphaeria maculans* (blackleg), *Fusarium oxysporum* (yellows or fusarium wilt), *Xanthomonas campestris* (black rot),

Brevicoryne brassicae (aphids), *Prodenia* spp. (cut worms), *Pieris rapae* (cabbage worms), and *Delia radicum* (cabbage root fly) infect *Brassica* and crucifers causing harmful diseases and damage [3, 11]. The utilization of pesticides to control these devastated diseases is harmful for human and environment. The issue has led to searching for alternative resources to control these diseases. To close this gap, disease-resistant *Brassica* varieties would be developed in future breeding programs in order to improve their conservation and agricultural production [3]. Hence, attention has been paid to wild *Brassica* genetic resources (repositories of resistance genes) to identify the genes conferring resistance and good agronomic traits including oil content [2, 3, 12–14]. Due to the strong self-incompatibility system, most *Brassica* crops are outbreeders with a high degree of heterozygosity in natural populations and open-pollinated crops [3, 9]. Better methods for characterizing those germplasm collections have also been developed to improve strategies for their biodiversity conservation and utilization in varietal improvement.

2. Genetic characterization of *Brassica* germplasm

Genetic diversity is defined as the variation of individual genotypes within and among species and is the raw material permitting species to adjust to a changing world [2, 3]. Knowledge of the amount and distribution of genetic variability within a species is important for establishing efficient conservation and breeding practices [3], whereas it provides plant breeders with options to develop, through selection and breeding, new and more productive crops that are resistant to diseases and pests and adapted to changing environments. It also provides information for domestication and designing sampling protocols [3]. Therefore, assessing genetic diversity is also essential for providing information for domestication, propagation, and breeding programs as well as conservation of plant genetic resources. Different techniques and markers have been successfully used for characterizing *Brassica* genetic resources [3]. These techniques include morphological, cytological, biochemical, and molecular markers. Physiological, biochemical, and molecular genetic techniques have also successfully applied in different plant species [15–31]. This work highlights the current knowledge of the application of physiological and genetic markers in the genus *Brassica* L. in order to understand its biology, diversity, conservation, and breeding as a basis for further research to develop disease-resistant and more productive crops. Breeding technologies and resistance to abiotic stresses in *Brassica* species are also discussed.

Author details

Mohamed A. El-Esawi[1,2*]

*Address all correspondence to: mohamed.elesawi@science.tanta.edu.eg

1 Botany Department, Faculty of Science, Tanta University, Tanta, Egypt

2 The Sainsbury Laboratory, University of Cambridge, Cambridge, United Kingdom

References

[1] Rakow G. Species origin and economic importance of *Brassica*. In: Pua EC, Douglas CJ, editors. Biotechnology in Agriculture and Forestry. Vol. 54. New York: Springer-Verlag Berlin Heidelberg; 2004. pp. 3-11

[2] Christopher GL, Andrew JR, Geraldine ACL, Clare JH, Jacqueline B, Gary B, German CS, David E. *Brassica* ASTRA: An integrated database for *Brassica* genomic research. Nucleic Acids Research. 2005;**1**(33):D656-D659

[3] El-Esawi MA. Taxonomic relationships and biochemical genetic characterization of *Brassica* resources: Towards a recent platform for germplasm improvement and utilization. Annual Research & Review in Biology. 2015;**8**(4):1-11

[4] El-Esawi MA. Genetic diversity and evolution of *Brassica* genetic resources: From morphology to novel genomic technologies—A review. Plant Genetic Resources and Characterization. 2017;**15**:388-399

[5] El-Esawi MA, Germaine K, Bourke P, Malone R. Genetic diversity and population structure of *Brassica oleracea* germplasm in Ireland using SSR markers. Comptes Rendus Biologies. 2016;**339**:133-140

[6] Zhao J. The genetics of phytate content and morphological traits in *Brassica rapa* [PhD thesis]. The Netherlands: Wageningen University; 2007

[7] Labana KS, Gupta ML. Importance and origin. In: Labana KS, Banga SS, Banga SK, editors. Breeding Oilseed Brassicas. Berlin, Germany: Springer, Verlag Press; 1993. pp. 1-20

[8] Fahey J, Talalay P. The role of crucifers in cancer chemoprotection. In: Gustine DL, Florens HE, editors. Phytochemicals and Health. Rockville, USA: American Society of Plant Physiologists; 1995. pp. 87-93

[9] King GJ. A white paper for the multinational *Brassica* genome project. 2015. Available online at http://www.brassica.info/info/publications/white_paper.php

[10] Faltusová Z, Kučera L, Ovesná J. Genetic diversity of *Brassica* oleracea var. capitata Gene Bank accessions assessed by AFLP. Electronic Journal of Biotechnology. 2011;**14**(3):1-10

[11] Relf D, McDaniel A. Cole Crops or Brassicas. Virginia Cooperative Extension, Publication Number 426-403. Petersburg, USA: Virginia State University; 2009

[12] Lázaro A, Auginagalde I. Genetic diversity in *Brassica oleracea* L. (Cruciferae) and wild relatives (2n = 18) using isozymes. Annals of Botany. 1998;**82**:821-828

[13] Warwick SI, Francis A, La Fleche J. Guide to Wild Germplasm of *Brassica* and Allied Crops (Tribe Brassiceae, Brassicaceae). Ottawa, Canada: Agriculture and agri-food Canada, Eastern Cereal and Oilseeds Research Centre; 2000

[14] Watson-Jones SJ, Maxted N, Ford-Lloyd BV. Population baseline data for monitoring genetic diversity loss for 2010: A case study for *Brassica* species in the UK. Biological Conservation. 2006;**132**:490-499

[15] Consentino L, Lambert S, Martino C, Jourdan N, Bouchet PE, Witczak J, Castello P, El-Esawi M, Corbineau F, d'Harlingue A, Ahmad M. Blue-light dependent reactive oxygen species formation by Arabidopsis cryptochrome may define a novel evolutionarily conserved signalling mechanism. New Phytologist. 2015;**206**:1450-1462

[16] Elansary HO, Szopa A, Kubica P, Ekiert H, Ali HM, Elshikh MS, et al. Bioactivities of traditional medicinal plants in Alexandria. Evidence-Based Complementary and Alternative Medicine. 2018;**2018**:1463579

[17] Elansary HO, Yessoufou K, Abdel-Hamid AME, El-Esawi MA, Ali HM, Elshikh MS. Seaweed extracts enhance Salam turfgrass performance during prolonged irrigation intervals and saline shock. Frontiers in Plant Science. 2017;**8**:830

[18] El-Esawi MA. Micropropagation technology and its applications for crop improvement. In: Anis M, Ahmad N, editors. Plant Tissue Culture: Propagation, Conservation and Crop Improvement. Singapore: Springer; 2016. pp. 523-545

[19] El-Esawi MA. Nonzygotic embryogenesis for plant development. In: Anis M, Ahmad N, editors. Plant Tissue Culture: Propagation, Conservation and Crop Improvement. Singapore: Springer; 2016. pp. 583-598

[20] El-Esawi MA. Somatic hybridization and microspore culture in *Brassica* improvement. In: Anis M, Ahmad N, editors. Plant Tissue Culture: Propagation, Conservation and Crop Improvement. Singapore: Springer; 2016. pp. 599-609

[21] El-Esawi MA. SSR analysis of genetic diversity and structure of the germplasm of faba bean (*Vicia faba* L.). Comptes Rendus Biologies. 2017;**340**:474-480

[22] El-Esawi MA, Sammour R. Karyological and phylogenetic studies in the genus *Lactuca* L. (Asteraceae). Cytologia. 2014;**79**:269-275

[23] El-Esawi M, Arthaut L, Jourdan N, d'Harlingue A, Martino C, Ahmad M. Blue-light induced biosynthesis of ROS contributes to the signaling mechanism of Arabidopsis cryptochrome. Scientific Reports. 2017;**7**:13875

[24] El-Esawi MA, Elansary HO, El-Shanhorey NA, Abdel-Hamid AME, Ali HM, Elshikh MS. Salicylic acid-regulated antioxidant mechanisms and gene expression enhance rosemary performance under saline conditions. Frontiers in Physiology. 2017;**8**:716

[25] El-Esawi MA, Elkelish A, Elansary HO, et al. Genetic transformation and hairy root induction enhance the antioxidant potential of *Lactuca serriola* L. Oxidative Medicine and Cellular Longevity. 2017; Article ID 5604746, 8 pages

[26] El-Esawi MA, Germaine K, Bourke P, Malone R. AFLP analysis of genetic diversity and phylogenetic relationships of *Brassica oleracea* in Ireland. Comptes Rendus Biologies. 2016;**133**:163-170

[27] El-Esawi M, Glascoe A, Engle D, Ritz T, Link J, Ahmad M. Cellular metabolites modulate *in vivo* signaling of *Arabidopsis* cryptochrome-1. Plant Signaling and Behaviour. 2015;**10**(9)

[28] El-Esawi MA, Mustafa A, Badr S, Sammour R. Isozyme analysis of genetic variability and population structure of *Lactuca* L. germplasm. Biochemical Systematic and Ecology. 2017;**70**:73-79

[29] El-Esawi MA, Witczak J, Abomohra A, Ali HM, Elshikh MS, Ahmad M. Analysis of the genetic diversity and population structure of Austrian and Belgian wheat germplasm within a regional context based on DArT markers. Genes. 2018;**9**(1):47

[30] Jourdan N, Martino C, El-Esawi M, Witczak J, Bouchet PE, d'Harlingue A, Ahmad M. Bluelight dependent ROS formation by Arabidopsis cryptochrome-2 may contribute towards its signaling role. Plant Signaling and Behaviour. 2015, 2015;**10**(8):e1042647

[31] Vwioko E, Adinkwu O, El-Esawi MA. Comparative physiological, biochemical and genetic responses to prolonged waterlogging stress in okra and maize given exogenous ethylene priming. Frontiers in Physiology. 2017;**8**:632

Chapter 2

Phytochemical Composition and Antioxidant Potential of *Brassica*

Haq Nawaz, Muhammad Aslam Shad and
Saima Muzaffar

Additional information is available at the end of the chapter

http://dx.doi.org/10.5772/intechopen.76120

Abstract

The edible parts of *Brassica* plants are a rich source of phytochemical compounds which possess strong antioxidant potential. These plants contain a variety of phytochemical compound including phenolics, polyphenols, phenolic acids, flavonoids, carotenoids (zeaxanthin, lutein, β-carotene), alkaloids, phytosterols chlorophyll, glucosinolates, terpenoids, and glycosides. These plants possess strong antioxidant potential in terms of metal reducing, metal chelating, lipid reducing and free radical scavenging activities. These also have a positive effect on the activity of antioxidant enzymes such as glutathione peroxidase, superoxide dismutase, catalase, and ascorbate peroxidase. Among various species of genus *Brassica* studied for their phytochemical composition and antioxidant activity, *Brassica oleracea* leaves, florets and seeds have better phytochemical and antioxidant profile. *Brassica juncea, Brassica napus, Brassica rapa* and *Brassica nigra* are also the phytochemical and antioxidant rich species of genus *Brassica*. The phytochemical profile and antioxidant potential of *Brassica* plants make them the preferable candidates for nutritional and pharmaceutical applications.

Keywords: antioxidant potential, antioxidant enzymes, *Brassica* plants, free radical scavenging capacity, bioactive phytochemicals, phytochemical composition

1. Introduction

Brassica is a genus of plants family *Cruciferae* also called *Brassicaceae* which consists of about 350 genera and almost 3500 species. *Brassica* is the most important of all the genera of this family. Most of the species this genus have worldwide importance due to their economic, nutritional, medicinal, and pharmaceutical value. These species are cultivated as vegetables, oilseed crops, animal forage and medicinal herbs throughout the world. Oilseed crops of *Brassica* produce 14% of the world's vegetable oil, the third most important source of edible oil after soybean and palm.

The genus *Brassica* is classified as:

Kingdom	Planta
Division	Tracheophyta
Subdivision	Spermatophyta
Class	Angiospermae
Subclass	Dicotyledonae
Order	Papaverales
Family	Cruciferae or Brassicaceae
Genus	*Brassica*

Some commonly used *Brassica* species of nutritional and medicinal importance are enlisted below [1]:

Species	Subspecies/var.	Common name
Brassica oleracea	Capitata *F. alba*	White Cabbage
	Capitata *F. rubra*	Red or purple cabbage
	Capitata L.	Green cabbage
	Italica	Italian broccoli, Chinese broccoli
	Gemmifera	Brussels sprouts
	Sabellica L.	Curly kale
	Acephala L.	Kale
	Alboglabra	Chinese kale, kailan
	Botrytis	Cauliflower, Italian cauliflower
	Sabauda	Savoy cabbage
	Gongylodes	Kohlrabi, stem turnip, Knol khol
	Costata	Portuguese cole, Tronchuda cabbage
Brassica juncea	Czern L.	Mustard, Indian mustard, Leaf mustard,
Brassica juncea	Coss L.,	Green mustard
Brassica juncea	Integrifolia	Korean leaf mustard, Multi-shoot mustard
Brassica rapa or.		
Brassica campestris	Rapifera L./Rapa L	Sarson, Turnip rape, Field mustard, Bird
		rape, canola, Turnip top.

	Pekinensis L.	Chinese cabbage
	Parachinesis	Chines cabbage, Choi sum, Sawi
Brassica napus	Napobrassica	Oilseed rape, rape, oilseed rape, Canola
Brassica carinata		Ethiopian rapeseed
Brassica nigra	Koch L.	Black mustard
	Viridis	Collards
Brassica juncea	Crispifolia	Curled mustard
	Rosularis	Tatsoi
Brassica hirta	*Sinapis alba*	White or yellow mustard
Brassica elongata		Elongated mustard
Brassica fruticulosa		Mediterranean cabbage
Brassica hilarionis		Hilarion's *Brassica*, St. Hilarion Lahanas
Brassica kaber		Wild mustard, Charlock, Field mustard
Brassica balearica		Mallorca cabbage
Brassica fruticulosa		Mediterranean cabbage.
Brassica hilarionis		St Hilarion cabbage.
Brassica rupestris		Brown mustard
Brassica tournefortii		Asian mustard
Brassica narinosa		Broad beaked mustard
Brassica geniculata		Hoary mustard
Brassica elongate		Elongated mustard
Brassica septiceps		Seven top turnip
Brassica perviridis		Tender green, mustard spinach

B. oleracea is the most important species of genus *Brassica* due to its cultivation, consumption and nutritional and medicinal value. The members of this species are commonly called as cabbage, kale, broccoli, cauliflower and Brussels sprouts. These are equally used as vegetables for human and forage for animals. *B. juncea, B. napus, B. nigra, B. napus, B. carinata and B. rapa* are the other commonly used species of this genus which are used as vegetables and a source of vegetable oil. The parts of *Brassica* plants used as food and medicine include root, shoot, stem, leaves, leaf buds, flower buds, florets, landraces, sprouts, inflorescence, seeds, seed oil, and callus. The *Brassica* plants are very rich and economical source of a variety of nutritional (carbohydrates, lipids, protein, vitamins, and minerals) and phytochemical components of medicinal value.

Species/subspecies	Phytochemical components and biological activity	Reference
B. oleracea Capitata *F. alba*	Leaves are rich source of phytochemicals including phenolics, phenolic acids, sophoroside-glucosides and vitamin C with good antioxidant activity in terms of PORS and ORAC.	[5, 34, 35]
B. oleracea Capitata L.	Leaves and flower buds contain phenolic acids, phenols, polyphenols, tannins, saponins, carotenoids (zeaxanthin, lutein, β-carotene), alkaloids, phenols, phytosterols and chlorophyll, glucosinolates, terpenoids flavonoids, glycosides, steroids, anthocyanins and aliphatic and aromatic amines. It shows antioxidant activity in terms of FRAP, ICA, LARC, hydroxyl and DPPH radical scavenging activities. Leaves possess antioxidant enzymes including POD, SOD, and CAT, inhibit DNA methylation, and prevent DNA damage and threats of cancer and cardiovascular diseases.	[6, 21, 36–41]
B. oleracea Capitata *F. rubra*	Leaves are rich in phytochemicals including phenolics, carotenoids (zeaxanthin, lutein, β-carotene) glucosinolates, anthocyanins and vitamin C with good antioxidant activity in terms of free radical scavenging capacity.	[15, 35, 40]
B. oleracea Italica	Florets and stem contain phenolics, phenolic acids, polyphenols, sophoroside-glucosides, flavonoids, alkaloids, steroids, phenols, tannins, saponins, glutathione, glucosinolates (glucoraphanin, glucobrassicin, neoglucobrassicin), terpenoids, coumarins, cumins, cardiac glycosides, xanthoproteins, glycosides, carotenoids (zeaxanthin, lutein, β-carotene), tocopherols, phytosterols, chlorophyll, free sugars and vitamin C, and possesses antioxidant activity. It possesses antioxidant enzymes including POD, SOD, and CAT. It inhibits DNA methylation and prevents DNA damage and threats of cancer and cardiovascular diseases. It also possesses Antiproliferative, neuroprotective, antidiabetic, and antigenotoxic activities.	[5, 21, 29, 42–50]
	Seeds also possess antioxidant activity (ABTS, DPPH and SOA radical scavenging activity).	[51]
B. oleracea Gemmifera	Leaves are rich in phytochemicals including phenolic acids, phenols, flavonoids, glucosinolates, thiocyanates, carotenoids (zeaxanthin, lutein, β-carotene), phytosterols and chlorophyll. It possesses antioxidant activity in terms of free radical scavenging capacity and antioxidant enzymes activity (POD, SOD, and CAT). It inhibits DNA methylation, prevent DNA damage and threats of cancer and cardiovascular diseases.	[35, 40]
B. oleracea Sabellica L.	Leaves contain phenolics, polyphenols, glucosinolate, sugars, flavonoid, and flavonoids glycoside and show antioxidant activity in terms of FRAP, DPPH radical scavenging activity	[38, 52]
B. oleracea Acephala L.	Leaves contain polyphenols, Vitamin C and carotenoids (β-carotene) and possess antioxidant activity (ABTS radical scavenging activity).	[53]
Alboglabra	Leaves contain phenolics, Polyphenols, Glucosinolate, and Carotenoids (zeaxanthin, lutein, b-carotene),	[40]
B. oleracea Botrytis	Florets and leaves contain phenolics, polyphenols, alkaloids, saponins, tannins, steroids, flavonoids, glucosinolates, volatiles, reducing sugars and vitamin C. The aqueous and ethanolic extracts of root and leaves show antioxidant activity in terms of Fe reducing, Cu reducing, and Fe^{2+} chelating activity, ORAC, and DPPH, ABTS, and SOA radical scavenging activity. Florets possess antioxidant enzymes including POD, SOD, and CAT. It inhibits DNA methylation, prevent DNA damage and threats of cancer and cardiovascular diseases. It also possesses thrombolytic and cytotoxic activities.	[10, 42, 47, 54–57]

Species/subspecies	Phytochemical components and biological activity	Reference
B. oleracea Sabauda	Leaves are rich in phytochemicals including phenolics, chlorophyll, and glucosinolate (sinigrin) with good antioxidant and pro-oxidant activity in terms of ABTS and DPPH radical scavenging capacity.	[7, 30, 35]
B. oleracea Gongylodes	The extracts of knobs in various solvents have been found to improve the antioxidant status of liver and kidneys of diabetic animals by increasing the SOD and CAT activities.	[21]
B. oleracea Costata	Seeds, sprouts, and leaves possess the ability to reduces hypochlorous acid, inhibit hydroxyl, SO, and DPPH radicals. These also show a concentration-dependent increase in the activity of antioxidant enzyme SOD.	[3, 4]
B. juncea L. Czern.	Leaves contain flavonoids, terpenoids, tannins, reducing sugars vitamin C, benzenepropanoic acid, n-eicosane, n-pentacosane and n-tetratetracontane. It enhances the activity of antioxidant enzymes including GPx, CAT, and APx. Seeds contain sinigrin, quercetin, catechin, sophoroside-glucosides and vitamin E and seed oil possesses antioxidant activity in terms of FRAP, Fe chelating and DPPH and SOA radical scavenging activity. It also possesses cytotoxic activity.	[5, 12, 13, 15, 28, 54, 58, 59]
B. juncea L. Coss	It contains phenolic compounds with antioxidant activity in terms of FRAP and DPPH radical scavenging activity.	[58]
B. juncea integrifolia	Germplasm contain glucosinolates (sinigrin gluconasturtin and progoitrin).	[16]
B. rapa L. Rapifera or *B. campestris*	Root, stem, leaves, and flowers contain phenolics including 3-p-coumaroylquinic, caffeic, ferulic and sinapic acids, kaempferol sophoroside-glucosides and organic acids including aconitic, citric, ketoglutaric, malic, shikimic and fumaric acids. Roots possess antioxidant activity in terms of FRSC, RP, ILPO, and DPPH and SOA radical scavenging capacity. It also possesses cytotoxic activity.	[4, 54, 60–62]
B. rapa L. Pekinensis	Leaves possess antioxidant activity in terms of Fe reducing, oxygen radical absorbing capacity, and are also active against DPPH and ABTS radicals.	[63]
B. rapa L. Parachinesis	Leaves contain phenolics, flavonoids, and anthocyanins possessing antioxidant activity in terms of DPPH radical scavenging activity.	[9]
B. napus Napobrassica	Root and leaves possess antioxidant activity in terms of FRAP, inhibit lipid peroxidation and increase the SOD and GPx activity.	[32]
B. nigra L. Koch	Leaves, Seeds and callus contain phenolics (gallic acid, catechin, epicatechin, myricetin, quercetin, and rutin), flavonoids, tannins, saponins, sinigrin, cyanogenic and cardiac glycosides, alkaloids, glutathione reducing sugar, phlobatannins and volatile oil and possess antioxidant and antiradical activity (ORAC, FRAP, and DPPH and ABTS radical scavenging capacity).	[11, 14, 22, 25, 64–66]

ABTS: 2, 2-azinobis-(3-ethylbenzothiazoline-6-sulphonic acid), APx ascorbate peroxidase, CAT: catalase, DPPH: 2, 2-diphenyl-1-picrylhydrazyl, FRAP: ferric reducing antioxidant power, FRSC: free radical scavenging capacity, GPx: glutathione peroxidase, ICA: iron chelating activity, ILPO: inhibition of lipid peroxidation, LARC: linoleic acid reduction capacity, ORAC: Oxygen radical absorbance capacity, POD: peroxidase, PORSC: peroxide radical scavenging capacity, RP: reducing power, SO: superoxide, SOA: superoxide anion, SOD: superoxide dismutase.

Table 1. Bioactive phytochemical components and biological activities of some commonly used ***Brassica*** species.

2. Phytochemical composition

2.1. Phytochemical quality

Phytochemicals are non-nutritious chemicals that are derived from plants and provide defense against diseases in humans. They are oxidation preventive and sweep out free radicals, the byproducts of biochemical processes. They provide safeguard against different neurological, cardiac and many other physiological ailments and protect important biomolecules from oxidative damage [2]. *Brassica* plants are the rich source of phytochemical compounds of medicinal importance. A large no of *Brassica* plants has been studied for their bioactive phytochemical components and antioxidant potential. The bioactive compounds and antioxidant potential of commonly used species of *Brassica* plants are given in **Table 1**. The bioactive phytochemical compounds commonly found in most of the *Brassica* species include polyphenols, phenolic acids, flavonoids, carotenoids (zeaxanthin, lutein, β-carotene), alkaloids, tannins, saponins, anthocyanins, phytosterols chlorophyll, glucosinolates, phytosteroids, terpenoids, glycosides, vitamin C, Vitamin E and aliphatic and aromatic amines [3–16]. *B. oleracea* var. Capitata, *B. oleracea* var. Italica, *B. oleracea* var. Botrytis, *B. juncea, B. rapa* and *B. nigra* contain a treasure of phytochemical compounds of medicinal and pharmaceutical importance. Due to the presence of these compounds, *Brassica* plants show biological activities against various diseases and have been found to effective in treating various diseases in human. The edible parts of these plants show antimicrobial, antibacterial, antidiabetic, antimalarial, antiaging, antiulcer, anti-hyperglycemic, anti-hyperlipidemic, anti-proliferative, neuroprotective, antidiabetic, anti-genotoxic and antioxidant activities [17–25].

2.2. Phytochemical content

The major phytochemical compounds quantitatively estimated in various species of *Brassica* include phenolics, flavonoids, ascorbic acid (Vit. C) glucosinolates, carotenoids, and tocopherols. **Tables 2 and 3** present the phytochemical content (total phenolic content: TPC, total flavonoid content: TFC, ascorbic acid content: AAC, total glucosinolate content: TGC, total

Species/ subspecies	Parts used	Extracting solvent	TPC (GAE)	TFC	AAC	References
B. oleracea Capitata F. Alba	Leaves	Ethanol, methanol, acetone	14.78–18.7 mg/g extract	4.12–8.80 mg QE/g extract		[67]
		70% methanol, phosphoric acid	20–29 mg/100 g fw		18–35 mg/100 g fw	[35]
	Terminal leaf buds	Water	43.87 mg/g			[68]
B. oleracea Capitata F. Rubra	Leaves	70% methanol	134–171 mg/100 g fw			[24]

Species/ subspecies	Parts used	Extracting solvent	TPC (GAE)	TFC	AAC	References
B. oleracea Capitata L.	Leaves	80% methanol	3.64 μM/g dw			[37]
	Leaves	Varying polarity solvents	34–520 mg/100 g dw		3.20–8.30 g/100 g extract	[41]
		Varying polarity solvents	402–556 mg/100 g fw			[6]
	Flower buds	80% methanol, phosphoric acid	4.14 mM/g dw		62–72 mg/100 g fw	[37]
	leaf buds	Water	53.85 mg/g			[68]
B. oleracea Italica	Floret	Ethanol, methanol, acetone	17.9–23.6 mg/g extract	12.5–17.5 mg CE/100 g		[67]
		Water	48.76 μg/ml extract	69.64 μg/ml extract	25.0–29.48 μg/ml extract	[46]
	Florets, Leaves	Methanol, phosphoric acid	533.6–740 mg/100 g	317–816 mg CE/100 g	298.6–474.7 mg/100 g	[47]
	Florets	Methanol	43–75 mg/kg dw		2.1–4.0 mg/kg dw	[29]
	Inflore-scence	Water	1.816 mg/g fw			[48]
B. oleracea Gemmifera	Sprouts	Ethanol, methanol, acetone	18.12–20.4 mg/g extract	12.1–15.4 mg CE/100 g		[67]
		70% methanol, phosphoric acid	133–140 mg/100 g fw		129–127 mg/100 g fw	[35]
B. oleracea Alboglabra	Leaves	Water	35.64 mg/ g dw	13.98 mg QE/g dw		[52]
	Edible portion	Ethanol	30.51–38.30 mg/ g extract	28.99–70.69 mg QE/g extract		[9]
B. oleracea Acephala L.	Edible Leaves	Ethanol	574.9 mg/100 g fw, 6.37 mM/100 g		62.27 mg/100 g fw	[53]
B. oleracea Botrytis	Edible floret	80% ethanol	782.43 mg/100 g dw	267.21 mg CE/100 g dw	769.23 mg/100 g	[69]
B. oleracea Botrytis Cimosa	Edible portion	Ethanol	2.24 mM/ g			
	Inflore-scence	Water	30.4 mg/g			[68]

Species/ subspecies	Parts used	Extracting solvent	TPC (GAE)	TFC	AAC	References
	Florets, leaves	Methanol	350–1345 μg/100 g	90–780 mg CE/100 g		[47]
		phosphoric acid			396–649 mg/100 g	[47]
B. oleracea Sabauda	Leaves	70% methanol, phosphoric acid	47–59 mg/100 g fw		49–51 mg/100 g fw	[35]
B. oleracea Capitata	Leaves	Methanol	102.71 mg/100 g fw			[60]
B. juncea L. Czern.	Leaves	Water			0.1 mg/g fw	[70]
	Leaf, stem	Hexane methanol water	3.01–3.85 mg/100 g sample			[58]
B. juncea L. Coss Sareptana	Leaf, stem	Hexane methanol water	14.12–19.78 mg/100 g sample			[58]
B. rapa Rapifera L.	Root	70% ethanol	0.21–2.59 g/100 g dw			[61]
		Water	5.640 mg/g			[68]
	Root, Shoot, Leaves	Methanol	30–78 mg/100 g fw	4.1–8.5 mg RE/g fw	0.13–0.25 mg/g	[71]
B. rapa Pekinensis L.	Leaves	75% Methanol	150–347 mg/100 g	61.9–328.70	7.04–13.68	[63]
B. rapa Parachinesis	Leaves	Ethanol	42.32–42.92 mg/g extract	49–133 mg QE/g extract		[9]
B. nigra L.	Seeds oil		142.86 μg/ml	23.43 μg CE/ml		[64]

AAC: Ascorbic acid content, CE: Catechin equivalent, dw: Dry weight, fw: Fresh weight, GAE: Gallic acid equivalent, QE: Quercetin equivalent, RE: Rutin equivalent, TFC: Total flavonoid content, TPC: Total phenolic content.

Table 2. Phenolic, flavonoids and ascorbic acid content of commonly used ***Brassica*** species.

carotenoid content: TCC, and total tocopherol content: TTC) of various extracts of some edible parts of commonly used *Brassica* species. The aqueous and organic extracts of the various parts of *Brassica* plants have been found to contain the considerable amounts of phenolics, flavonoids, carotenoids, ascorbic acid, and tocopherols which advocate the suitability of *Brassica* plants for pharmaceutical applications. Among *Brassica* species, *B. oleracea* var. Capitata, *B. oleracea* var. Italica, and *B. juncea*, *B. rapa* are high in phenolics, flavonoids and carotenoids.

Species/subspecies	Parts used	Extracting solvent	TGC	TCC	TTC mg/100 g fw	References
B. oleracea Capitata F. Alba	Leaves	Hexane		4.35–10.07 mg/100 g fw	0.008–0.22	[35]
	Terminal leaf buds	Water		4.33 mg/g		[68]
B. oleracea Capitata L.	Leaves, Flower buds	80% Methanol		0.28–12.51 μM/g dw		[37]
B. oleracea Capitata F. Rubra	Leaves	Hexane		2.73–2.80 mg/100 g fw	0.61–0.11	[35]
	Terminal leaf buds	Water		4.35 mg/g		[68]
B. oleracea Italica	Florets, Leaves	Methanol	2.12–9.66 μM/g dw			[47]
B. oleracea Gemmifera	Sprouts	Hexane		2.31–2.6 mg/100 g fw	0.545–0.83	[35]
B. oleracea Botrytis Cimosa	Edible portion	Acetone, petroleum ether		126.22 mg/100 g dw		[69]
	Inflore-scence	Water		2.62 mg/g		[68]
	Florets, leaves	Methanol	1.97–8.80 μM/g dw			[47]
B. oleracea Sabauda	Leaves	Hexane		5.55–6.25 mg/100 g fw	0.011–0.078	[35]
B. oleracea Capitate var. aabuada	Leaves	Methanol	195.22 μM/100 g fw			[7]
B. oleracea Gongylodes	Stem		20.69 mg/g	0.79 mg/g		[68]
B. rapa Rapifera L.	Root	Water		2.04 mg/g		[68]
B. rapa Pekinensis L.	Leaves	75% Methanol		3.93–18.87		[63]

TCC: Total carotenoid content, TGC: Total glucosinolate content, TTC: Total tocopherol content.

Table 3. Glucosinolate, total carotenoids and tocopherol content of commonly used ***Brassica*** species.

3. Antioxidant potential

Antioxidants are the compounds which prevent the oxidation of the biomolecules by reducing the oxidizing agents and being self-oxidized. These compounds have the ability to scavenge the free radicals produced during the redox reactions occurring in the living and nonliving systems and prevent the free radical chain reactions. In this way, the antioxidant compounds minimize the oxidative stress and prevent the oxidative damage to food materials and living organisms. *Brassica* plants are known to possess antioxidant properties due to the presence of antioxidant phytochemicals mainly the polyphenols, flavonoids and ascorbic acid. Most of these phytochemical compounds act as antioxidants due to their hydrogen donating and reducing abilities. Polyphenols are the phytochemicals which act as metal ion chelators and interfere with oxidation reactions including lipid peroxidation by donating the proton to free radicals. Phenoxy radicals are relatively stable to stop the oxidation chain reaction. Therefore, they stop the initiation of new oxidation chain reaction and terminate the propagation routs by capturing free radicals [26]. Polyphenols are used for the treatment of hypertension, vascular fragility, allergies and hypercholesterolemia due to their antimicrobials, antiulcer, antidiarrheal, and anti-inflammatory activities. Flavonoids possess metal ion chelating and free radical scavenging potential [27]. These phytochemicals comprise a vast antioxidant, antiproliferative and inhibitory action on inflammatory cells especially mast cells. Ascorbic acid is a water-soluble vitamin which possesses strong antioxidant potential and protects against oxidative damage.

The antioxidant activities of various extracts of some edible parts of commonly used *Brassica* species are presented in **Tables 4** and **5**. The *Brassica* plants have been found to possess metal

Species/subspecies	Parts used	Extracting solvent	TAOA	FRAP	ICA	References
B. oleracea Capitata L.	Leaves	80% Methanol		18.3 μM TE/g dw		[72]
		Series of solvents	574 g GAE/100 g dw			[41]
	Flower buds	80% methanol		15.37 μM TE/g dw		[37]
B. oleracea Italica	Sprouts		74.48–93.2%	35–75 g Fe^{2+}E/kg dw		[29]
	Inflore-scence	Water		0.998 mM $FeSO_4$/g fw		[48]
B. juncea L. Czern.	Seed oil	Ethanol, hexane			55.15%	[13]
	Leaf, stem	Hexane methanol water		2.25–3.12 mM $FeSO_4$/100 g sample		[58]
B. juncea L. Coss	Leaf, stem	Hexane methanol water	3.23–7.75 mM $FeSO_4$/100 g sample			[58]
B. rapa Rapifera L.			1.68 mM/L			[31]

Species/subspecies	Parts used	Extracting solvent	TAOA	FRAP	ICA	References
B. rapa Pekinensis L.			87–714.5 μM TE			[63]
B. napus Napobrassica	Leaves, root			0.91–2.31 Units		[32]
B. nigra L.	Seed oil			23.85%		[64]

FRAP: Ferric reducing antioxidant power, GAE: Gallic acid equivalent, ICA: Iron chelating activity, TAOA: Total antioxidant activity, TE: Trolox equivalent.

Table 4. Total antioxidant activity, metal reducing and metal chelating ability of commonly used ***Brassica*** species.

Species/subspecies	Parts used	Extracting solvent	DPPH·	SOA·	ABTS·	References
B. oleracea Capitata F. Alba		Ethanol, methanol, acetone	IC_{50}: 1.01–1.40 mg/ml			[67]
		70% methanol	0.77–1.0 μM AAE/g fw	IC_{50}: 4.35–10.07 mg/ml	1.34–1.8 μM TE/g fw	[35]
B. oleracea Capitata F. Rubra		70% methanol	6.76–9.19 μM AAE/g fw	IC_{50}: 2.73–2.80 mg/ml	9.8–12.6 μM TE/g fw	[35]
B. oleracea Capitata L.	Leaves	80% methanol	14.94 μM TE/g dw		24.78 μM TE/g dw	[37]
		Series of solvents	IC_{50}: 0.006–0.16 mg/ml			[41]
		Series of solvents	59.18–75.65% IC_{50}: 4.2–8.7 μg/ml			[6]
	Flower buds	80% Methanol	12.51 μM TE/g dw		25.16 μM TE/g dw	[37]
	Leaves	Ethanol	7.316 μM AAE/g fw			[39]
		Water	15.14 M AAE/g fw			[39]
B. oleracea Italica	Floret	Ethanol, methanol, acetone	IC_{50}: 0.71–1.35 mg/ml			[67]
		Water	47.93–85.40%			[46]
	Florets leaves	Methanol	IC_{50}: 2.27 mg/ml			[47]
	Inflore-scence	Water	EC_{50}: 0.25 mg/ml			[48]
B. oleracea Gemmifera		Ethanol, methanol, acetone	IC_{50}: 0.8–1.22 mg/ml			[67]
		70% methanol	3.90–5.98 μM AAE/g fw	IC_{50}: 2.31–2.60 mg/ml	5.85–7.04 μM TE/g fw	[35]

Species/subspecies	Parts used	Extracting solvent	DPPH·	SOA·	ABTS·	References
B. oleracea Alboglabra	Leaves	Water	IC_{50}: 18 μg/ml			[52]
		Ethanol	1.26–2.72% IC_{50}: 0.90–0.99 mg/ml			[9]
B. oleracea Botrytis	Florets	80% ethanol	68.91%			[69]
	Seed	DCM	IC_{50}: 1.51–2.75 mg/ml	IC_{50}: 0.17–0.26 mg/ml		[54]
B. oleracea Botrytis Cimosa	Edible portion	Ethanol	EC_{50}: 6.51 mg/l			[8]
B. oleracea Sabauda		70% methanol	1.38–1.68 μM AAE/g fw	IC_{50}: 5.55–6.25 mg/ml	2.89–3.74 μM TE/g fw	[35]
B. oleracea Acephala	Edible leaves	Ethanol	IC_{50}: 1.53 mg/ml		33.22 μM TE/g fw	[8, 53]
B. juncea L. Czern	Seed	Hexane	40.2–70.2%			[13]
		DCM	IC_{50}: 2.76–5.79 mg/ml	IC_{50}: 0.059–0.46 mg/ml		[54]
		Hexane methanol water	4.23–6.41 mM TE/100 g sample			[58]
B. juncea L. Coss		Hexane methanol water	6.86–8.18 mM TE/100 g sample			[58]
B. rapa Rapifera L.	Root	70% ethanol	IC_{50}: 0.23–2.00 mg/ml			[61]
	Root Shoot Leaves	Methanol	13–26%			[71]
	Root aerial parts	70% ethanol	11.11–86.3%			[62]
	Seed	DCM	IC_{50}: 2.78–5.92 mg/ml	IC_{50}: 0.003–0.03 mg/ml		[54]
B. rapa Pekinensis L.	Leaves	75% methanol	92–239 μM TE		175–393 μM TE	[63]
B. rapa Parachinesis	Leaves	Ethanol	5.5–6.26% IC_{50}: 0.55–1.01 mg/ml			[9]
B. nigra L.	Oilseed	Ethanol	89.25%			[64]
	Leaves	Ethanol	5.09–68.08%			[22]

AAE: Ascorbic acid equivalent, ABTS·: DPPH: EC_{50}: Effective concentration required for 50% inhibition, IC_{50}: Inhibitory concentration required for 50% inhibition, SOA: Superoxide anion radical, TE: Trolox equivalent.

Table 5. Free radical scavenging potential of commonly used ***Brassica*** species.

Species/subspecies	GPx	SOD	CAT	HO	APx	References
B. oleracea Gongylodes		41.26–42.35 U/mg protein (liver), 34.43–39.38-U/mg protein (kidney)	42.06–43.70 U, (Liver) 5.50–4.59 U (kidney)			[21]
B. juncea L. Czern.	$1.58x10^3$ U/mg GSH utilized/min/mg protein		3.75 μM H_2O_2 disposed/min/g protein	0.05–0.32 μM biliverdin reduced/min/mg protein)	0.52–0.61 mM APx oxidized/min/mg protein,	[33]
B. rapa Rapifera L.	6981 U/L	220 U/ml			95.23 μM/ml	[31]
B. napus Napobrassica	4.18–19.92 U/mg protein	66.80–202.30 U/mg protein				[32]

APx: ascorbate peroxidase, CAT: Catalase, GPx: Glutathione peroxidase, GSH: Glutathione, HO: Heme oxygenase, SOD: Superoxide dismutase.

Table 6. Antioxidant enzyme activities of commonly used ***Brassica*** species.

reducing, metal chelating, lipid reducing and free radical scavenging activities [24, 28–30]. These also possess antioxidant enzyme activities as these have been found to enhance the activities of some antioxidant enzymes including glutathione peroxidase, superoxide dismutase, catalase, heme oxygenase and ascorbate peroxidase [21, 31–33] (**Table 6**). *B. oleracea* plants have been studied most for their antioxidant activities among the *Brassica* species and found to possess strong antioxidant potential in terms of reducing power and free radical scavenging capacity. The strong antioxidant potential of *Brassica* plants highlights their medicinal and therapeutic importance.

4. Factors affecting the antioxidant activity of *Brassica* plants

Antioxidant activity of *Brassica* plants has been studied to be effected by various factors including solvent polarity, extraction time, temperature, cooking methods and nutritional and environment stress (**Table 7**). The increase in the polarity of the extracting solvent, extraction time and salinity stress has resulted in an increase in the antioxidant activity of *Brassica* plants. However, an increase in the temperature results in a reduction in the antioxidant potential of these plants. The steam boiling and microwave cooking methods result in a time-dependent decrease in the phytochemical content and antioxidant activity while water boiling, water blanching, steam boiling, steam blanching, microwave heating and stir-frying result in the reduction of antioxidant potential of *Brassica* vegetables.

Factors	Effects	References
Solvent polarity	Antioxidant activity increases with increasing the polarity of extracting solvent.	[61]
Extraction/ treatment Time	Increase in extraction time resulted in an increase in phytochemical content and antioxidant activity.	[41]
Temperature	High temperature resulted in a rapid decrease in flavonoid content of *B. oleracea* var. Italica.	[73]
Cooking method	Steam boiling and microwave cooking showed a time-dependent decrease in phytochemical content and antioxidant activity of green broccoli. Water boiling, water blanching, steam boiling, steam blanching, microwave heating and stir-frying resulted in the reduction of antioxidant potential of cauliflower.	[46, 69]
Salinity stress	Extracts of *B. juncea* L. under salinity stress have been found to be helpful in decreasing the oxidative stress by increasing the activity of activity of antioxidant enzymes.	[33]

Table 7. Factors affecting the phytochemical composition and antioxidant activity of some commonly used ***Brassica*** species.

5. Conclusion

The edible of *Brassica* plants have been found to be a rich source of phytochemical compounds which possess strong antioxidant potential. These plants possess strong antioxidant potential in terms of metal reducing, metal chelating, lipid reducing and free radical scavenging and antioxidant enzymes activities. *Brassica oleracea* has been found to possess better phytochemical and antioxidant profile among *Brassica* plants. *Brassica juncea, Brassica napus, Brassica rapa* and *Brassica nigra* are also phytochemical and antioxidant rich species of genus *Brassica*. The considerable amount of phytochemicals and antioxidant potential make the *Brassica* plants the preferable candidates for nutritional and pharmaceutical applications.

Conflict of interest

I confirm that there are no conflicts of interest.

Author details

Haq Nawaz[1]*, Muhammad Aslam Shad[1] and Saima Muzaffar[2]

*Address all correspondence to: haqnawaz@bzu.edu.pk

1 Department of Biochemistry, Bahuddin Zakariya University, Multan, Pakistan

2 Institute of Chemical Sciences, Bahuddin Zakariya University, Multan, Pakistan

References

[1] Genus *Brassica* [Internet]. Worldw. Veg. [cited 2018 Feb 4]. Available from: http://theworldwidevegetables.weebly.com/genus-*Brassica*.html

[2] Uttara B, Singh AV, Zamboni P, Mahajan RT. Oxidative stress and neurodegenerative diseases: A review of upstream and downstream antioxidant therapeutic options. Current Neuropharmacology. 2009;**7**:65-74

[3] Ferreres F, Valentão P, Llorach R, Pinheiro C, Cardoso L, Pereira JA, et al. Phenolic compounds in external leaves of tronchuda cabbage (*Brassica oleracea* L. var. costata DC). Journal of Agricultural and Food Chemistry. 2005;**53**:2901-2907

[4] Sousa C, Valentâo P, Pereira DM, Taveira M, Ferreres F, Pereira JA, et al. Phytochemical and antioxidant characterization of *Brassica oleracea* var. Costata extracts. Recent Progress in Medical Plants. 2009;**24**:311-339

[5] Cartea ME, Francisco M, Soengas P, Velasco P. Phenolic compounds in *Brassica* vegetables. Molecules. 2010;**16**:251-280

[6] Ahmed MF, Rao AS, Ahemad SR, Ibrahim M. Phytochemical studies and antioxidant activities of *Brassica oleracea* L. Var. Capitata. International Journal of Pharmacy and Pharmaceutical Sciences. 2012;**4**:374-378

[7] Fernández León AM, Lozano Ruiz M, González Gómez D, Ayuso Yuste MC, Fernández León MF. Bioactive compounds content and total antioxidant activity of two savoy cabbages. 2014

[8] Fratianni F, Cardinale F, Cozzolino A, Granese T, Pepe S, Riccardi R, et al. Polyphenol composition and antioxidant activity of two autochthonous Brassicaceae of the Campania region, southern Italy. Food and Nutrition Sciences. 2014;**5**:66

[9] Unal K, Susanti D, Taher M. Polyphenol content and antioxidant capacity in organically and conventionally grown vegetables. Journal of Coast Life Medicine. 2014;**2**:864-871

[10] Kamal AM, Chowdhury KAA, Shill LK, Hossain MR, Islam N, Anaytulla IA, et al. Phytochemical screening, cytotoxic and thrombolytic activity of extract of *Brassica oleracea* flower (cauliflower). Global Journal of Pharmacology. 2015;**9**:115-120

[11] Danlami U, Orishadipe Abayomi T, Lawal DR. Phytochemical, nutritional and antimicrobial evaluations of the aqueous extract of *Brassica Nigra* (Brassicaceae) seeds. American Journal of Applied Chemistry. 2016;**4**:161-163

[12] Sharma A, Kumar V, Kanwar MK, Thukral AK, Bhardwaj R. Phytochemical profiling of the leaves of *Brassica* juncea L. using GC-MS. International Food Research Journal. 2017:24

[13] Singh Y, Malik CP. Phenols and their antioxidant activity in *Brassica juncea* seedlings growing under HgCl2 stress. Journal of Microbiology and Biotechnology Research. 2017;**1**:124-130

[14] Al Shahawany AW, Al Hattab ZN, Al Tahhan SF. Qualitative and quantitative analysis of Sinigrin in different parts in vitro and in vivo of *Brassica nigra* plants. Biomedicine. 2016;**4**:19-24

[15] Chauhan ES, Tiwari A, Singh A. Phytochemical screening of red cabbage (*Brassica oleracea*) powder and juice-a comparative study. Journal of Medicinal Plants. 2016;**4**:196-199

[16] Kim HW, Ko HC, Baek HJ, Cho SM, Jang HH, Lee YM, et al. Identification and quantification of glucosinolates in Korean leaf mustard germplasm (*Brassica juncea* var. integrifolia) by liquid chromatography–electrospray ionization/tandem mass spectrometry. European Food Research and Technology. 2016;**242**:1479-1484

[17] Chen J, Zhang J, Xiang Y, Xiang L, Liu Y, He X, et al. Extracts of Tsai tai (*Brassica chinensis*): Enhanced antioxidant activity and anti-aging effects both in vitro and in *Caenorhabditis elegans*. Food & Function. 2016;**7**:943-952

[18] Suresh S, Waly MI, Guizani N, Rahman MS. Broccoli (*Brassica oleracea*) extract combats Streptozotocin-induced diabetes and oxidative stress in rats. The FASEB Journal. 2016;**30**:404-406

[19] Wang W, Wang X, Ye H, Hu B, Zhou L, Jabbar S, et al. Optimization of extraction, characterization and antioxidant activity of polysaccharides from *Brassica rapa* L. International Journal of Biological Macromolecules. 2016;**82**:979-988

[20] Soengas P, Sotelo T, Velasco P, Cartea ME. Antioxidant properties of *Brassica* vegetables. Functional Plant Science and Biotechnology. 2011;**5**:43-55

[21] Sharma I, Aaradhya M, Kodikonda M, Naik PR. Antihyperglycemic, antihyperlipidemic and antioxidant activity of phenolic rich extract of *Brassica oleraceae* var gongylodes on streptozotocin induced Wistar rats. Springerplus. 2015;**4**:212

[22] Tripathi A, Punekar R, Jain V, Tyagi CK, Chandekar A, Vyas A. Antioxidant and antiulcer potential on leaves of *Brassica nigra* L. against gastric ulcer. International Journal of Phytomedicine. 2017;**9**:144-150

[23] Muluye AB, Melese E, Adinew GM. Antimalarial activity of 80% methanolic extract of *Brassica nigra* (L.) Koch. (*Brassicaceae*) seeds against Plasmodium berghei infection in mice. BMC Complementary and Alternative Medicine. 2015;**15**:367

[24] Simlai A, Chatterjee K, Roy A. A comparative study on antioxidant potentials of some leafy vegetables consumed widely in India. Journal of Food Biochemistry. 2014;**38**:365-373

[25] Obi RK, Nwanebu FC, Ndubuisi UU, Orji NM. Antibacterial qualities and phytochemical screening of the oils of Curcubita pepo and *Brassica nigra*. Journal of Medicinal Plants Research. 2009;**3**:429-432

[26] Mandal SM, Chakraborty D, Dey S. Phenolic acids act as signaling molecules in plant-microbe symbioses. Plant Signaling & Behavior. 2010;**5**:359-368

[27] Chawla S, Saxena A, Seshadri S. In-vitro availability of iron in various green leafy vegetables. Journal of the Science of Food and Agriculture. 1988;**46**:125-127

[28] Kumari N, Avtar R, Thakral BSN. Antioxidant potential in seed meal of different Indian mustard genotypes. Journal of Oilseed *Brassica*. 2016;**1**:63-67

[29] Nicoletto C, Santagata S, Pino S, Sambo P. Antioxidant characterization of different italian broccoli landraces. Horticultura Brasileira. 2016;**34**:74-79

[30] Quassinti L, Gianfranceschi G, Lupidi G, Miano A, Bramucci M. Antioxidant and pro-oxidant activities of savoy cabbage (*Brassica oleracea* L. Var. Sabauda) sprout extracts. Journal of Food Biochemistry. 2016;**40**:542-549

[31] Gul S, Ahmed S, Gul H, Shad KF, Zia-Ul-Haq M, Badiu D. The antioxidant potential of *Brassica rapa* L. on glutathione peroxidase, superoxide dismutase enzymes and total antioxidant status. Revista Romana de Medicina de Laborator. 2013;**21**:161-169

[32] Jovičić D, Vasin J, Nikolić Z, Petrović G, Tamnidžić G, Ignjatov M, et al. Antioxidant capacity of oilseed rape (*Brassica napus*) in different soil types. Turkish Journal of Agriculture and Forestry. 2017;**41**:463-471

[33] Verma K, Dixit S, Shekhawat GS, Alam A. Antioxidant activity of heme oxygenase 1 in *Brassica juncea* (L.) Czern.(Indian mustard) under salt stress. Turkish Journal of Biology. 2015;**39**:540-549

[34] Podsędek A. Natural antioxidants and antioxidant capacity of *Brassica* vegetables: A review. LWT-Food Science Technology. 2007;**40**:1-11

[35] Sosnowska D, Redzynia M, Anders B. Antioxidant capacity and content of *Brassica oleracea* dietary antioxidants. International Journal of Food Science and Technology. 2006;**41**:49-58

[36] Ogbede S, Saidu A, Kabiru A. Phytochemical compositions, Antihyperlipidemic and Hepatoprotective effects of *Brassica oleracea* Var. Capitata L. leaf extracts on triton-induced Hyperlipidemic rats. International Journal of Medical Science and Clinical Invention. 2014;**1**:345-351

[37] Sotelo T, Cartea ME, Velasco P, Soengas P. Identification of antioxidant capacity-related QTLs in *Brassica oleracea*. PLoS One. 2014;**9**:e107290

[38] Grønbæk M. Effects of cultivation strategies on phytochemicals and sensory properties of cabbage (*Brassica oleracea L. var. capitata L.*) and curly kale (*Brassica oleracea* L. var. sabellica L.). Aarhus University, Department of Food Science; 2014

[39] Thaipratum R. Evaluation of antioxidant activities of cabbage (*Brassica oleracea* L. var. capitata L.). World Academy of Science, Engineering and Technology International Journal of Biology and Biomolecular Agricultural Food Biotechnology Engineering. 2014;**8**:591-593

[40] Hedges LJ, Lister CE. Nutritional Attributes of Brassica Vegetables. Crop Food Res Confid Rep. 2006

[41] Nawaz H, Shad MA, Rauf A. Optimization of extraction yield and antioxidant properties of *Brassica oleracea* Convar Capitata Var L. leaf extracts. Food Chemistry. 2018;**242**:182-187

[42] Sharma P, Kapoor S. Biopharmaceutical aspects of *Brassica* vegetables. Journal of Pharmacognosy and Phytochemistry. 2015;**4**

[43] Fulltext [Internet]. [cited 2018 Jan 29]. Available from: https://www.researchgate.net/profile/Carolyn_Lister/publication/268516193_Nutritional_attributes_of_Brassica_vegetables/links/546e86de0cf29806ec2eb695.pdf

[44] Miraj S. Broccoli (*Brassica oleracea* var. Italica): Potential candidate in the health management. Der Pharmacia Lettre. 2016;**8**:61-65

[45] Renaud EN, van Bueren ETL, Myers JR, Paulo MJ, van Eeuwijk FA, Zhu N, et al. Variation in broccoli cultivar phytochemical content under organic and conventional management systems: Implications in breeding for nutrition. PLoS One 2014;**9**:e95683

[46] Porter Y. Antioxidant properties of green broccoli and purple-sprouting broccoli under different cooking conditions. Bioscience Horizon. 2012;**5**:hzs004

[47] Bhandari SR, Kwak J-H. Seasonal variation in phytochemicals and antioxidant activities in different tissues of various broccoli cultivars. African Journal of Biotechnology. 2014:13

[48] Wu H, Zhu J, Yang L, Wang R, Wang C. Ultrasonic-assisted enzymatic extraction of phenolics from broccoli (*Brassica oleracea* L. var. italica) inflorescences and evaluation of antioxidant activity in vitro. Food Science and Technology International. 2015;**21**:306-319

[49] Singh B, Chaturvedi S, Walia S, Kaushik G, Thakur S. Antioxidant potential of broccoli stalk: A preliminary investigation. Mediterranean Journal of Nutrition and Metabolism. 2011;**4**:227-230

[50] Shah MA, Sarker MMR, Gousuddin M. Antidiabetic potential of *Brassica oleracea* Var. Italica in type 2 diabetic Sprague dawley (sd) rats. International Journal of Pharmacognosy and Phytochemistry Research. 2016;**8**:462-469

[51] Ligen Z, Yuanfeng W, Yuke S, Lei Z, Mupunga J, Jianwei M, et al. Broccoli seed extracts but not sulforaphane have strong free radical scavenging activities. International Journal of Food Science and Technology. 2017;**52**:2374-2381

[52] Agarwal A, Raj N, Chaturvedi N. A comparative study on proximate and antioxidant activity of *Brassica oleracea* (kale) and *Spinacea oleracea* (spinach) leaves. International Journal of Advanced Research Biological Sciences. 2017;**4**:22-29

[53] Sikora E, Bodziarczyk I. Composition and antioxidant activity of kale (*Brassica* oleracea L. var. acephala) raw and cooked. Acta Scientiarum Polonorum. Technologia Alimentaria. 2012;**11**:239-248

[54] Chaudhary A, Choudhary S, Sharma U, Vig AP, Arora S. In vitro evaluation of *Brassica* sprouts for its antioxidant and Antiproliferative potential. Indian Journal of Pharmaceutical Sciences. 2016;**78**:615-623

[55] Lo Scalzo R, Picchi V, Migliori CA, Campanelli G, Leteo F, Ferrari V, et al. Variations in the phytochemical contents and antioxidant capacity of organically and conventionally grown Italian cauliflower (*Brassica oleracea* L. subsp. botrytis): Results from a three-year field study. Journal of Agricultural and Food Chemistry. 2013;**61**:10335-10344

[56] Cabello-Hurtado F, Gicquel M, Esnault M-A. Evaluation of the antioxidant potential of cauliflower (*Brassica oleracea*) from a glucosinolate content perspective. Food Chemistry. 2012;**132**:1003-1009

[57] Köksal E, Gülçin İ. Antioxidant activity of cauliflower (*Brassica oleracea* L.). Turkish Journal of Agriculture and Forestry. 2008;**32**:65-78

[58] Puangkam K, Muanghorm W, Konsue N. Stability of bioactive compounds and antioxidant activity of Thai cruciferous vegetables during in vitro digestion. Current Research Nutrition in Food Science Journal. 2017;**5**:100-108

[59] Parikh H, Khanna A. Pharmacognosy and phytochemical analysis of *Brassica juncea* seeds. Pharmacognosy Journal. 2014;**6**

[60] Fernandes F, Valentão P, Sousa C, Pereira JA, Seabra RM, Andrade PB. Chemical and antioxidative assessment of dietary turnip (*Brassica rapa* var. rapa L.). Food Chemistry. 2007;**105**:1003-1010

[61] Ryu JP, Kim DC, In M-J, Chae HJ, Lee SD. Antioxidant potential of ethanol extract of *Brassica rapa* L. root. Journal of Medicinal Plants Research. 2012;**6**:1581-1584

[62] Beltagy AM. Investigation of new antimicrobial and antioxidant activities of *Brassica rapa* L. International Journal of Pharmacy and Pharmaceutical Sciences. 2014;**6**:84-88

[63] Seong G-U, Hwang I-W, Chung S-K. Antioxidant capacities and polyphenolics of Chinese cabbage (*Brassica rapa* L. ssp. Pekinensis) leaves. Food Chemistry. 2016;**199**:612-618

[64] Olgun Ç, Özkan OE, Güney B, Pattabanoglu ES, Güney K, Gür M. Chemical composition and antimicrobial activity in cold press oil of fennel, Anise, white and black mustard seeds. Indian Journal of Pharmaceutical Educational Research. 2017;**51**:S200-S204

[65] Kumar M, Sharma S, Vasudeva N. In vivo assessment of antihyperglycemic and antioxidant activity from oil of seeds of *Brassica nigra* in streptozotocin induced diabetic rats. Advanced Pharmaceutical Bulletin. 2013;**3**:359

[66] Lee YH, Choo C, Waisundara VY. Determination of the Total antioxidant capacity and quantification of phenolic compounds of different solvent extracts of black mustard seeds (*Brassica nigra*). International Journal of Food Properties. 2015;**18**:2500-2507

[67] Jaiswal AK, Abu-Ghannam N, Gupta S. A comparative study on the polyphenolic content, antibacterial activity and antioxidant capacity of different solvent extracts of *Brassica oleracea* vegetables. International Journal of Food Science and Technology. 2012;**47**:223-231

[68] Anitha T. Studies on Invitro antioxidant properties of *Brassica* vegetables. International Journal of Pharmaceutical, Chemical and Biological Sciences. 2014;**4**

[69] Ahmed FA, Ali RF. Bioactive compounds and antioxidant activity of fresh and processed white cauliflower. BioMed Research International. 2013;**2013**

[70] Chauhan PK, Jaryal M, Kumari K, Singh M. Phytochemical and in vitro antioxidant potential of aqueous leaf extracts of *Brassica juncea* and Coriandrum sativum. International Journal of Pharmaceutical Sciences and Research. 2012;**3**:2862

[71] Iqbal S, Younas U, Chan KW, Saeed Z, Shaheen MA, Akhtar N, et al. Growth and antioxidant response of *Brassica rapa* var. rapa L.(turnip) irrigated with different compositions of paper and board mill (PBM) effluent. Chemosphere. 2013;**91**:1196-1202

[72] Fulltext [Internet]. [cited 2018 Jan 29]. Available from: http://journals.plos.org/plosone/article?id=10.1371/journal.pone.0107290

[73] Balouchi Z, Peyvast G-A, Ghasemnezhad M, Saadatian M. Changes of antioxidant compounds of broccoli (*Brassica oleracea* l. var. Italica) during storage at low and high temperatures. Journal of Horticulture, Biology and Environment. 2011;**2**(2):193-212

Chapter 3

Spatial and Temporal Assessment of *Brassica napus* L. Maintaining Genetic Diversity and Gene Flow Potential: An Empirical Evaluation

Vladimir Meglič and Barbara Pipan

Additional information is available at the end of the chapter

http://dx.doi.org/10.5772/intechopen.74570

Abstract

Unpredicted persistence of all forms of *B. napus* present in the agro-ecosystem is the most common consequence of preservation and self-recruitment of seeds originating from soil seed bank. In nature, spontaneous intra- and inter-specific hybridization of *B. napus* is possible with sexually compatible species from the Brassicaceae family. The aim of this chapter is (a) to identify the distribution pattern and population dynamics of volunteers and feral populations along statistical regions in Slovenia; (b) to assess the global diversity of naturally appearing *B. napus* plants; (c) to evaluate the genetic differentiation between volunteers and feral populations; (d) to obtain the spatial and temporal distribution of spontaneous pollination potential and estimation of gene flow conservation; (e) to find the empirically assigned out-crossing rate of *B. napus* under a fragmented landscape structure, during 4-year monitoring; and (f) to observe that ecologically, evolutionary, and agronomically oriented studies could be conducted at the DNA level using short sequence repeat (SSR) markers. In total, we collected 261 samples of volunteer and feral populations. Our results showed that alleles from both volunteer and feral populations were distributed in three genetic clusters with relatively similar levels of diversity. Naturally occurring out-crossing rate is 13.71%. The global Mantel correlation coefficient of genetic and spatial relatedness between genotypes is 0.044.

Keywords: *Brassica napus* L., feral populations, volunteers, spontaneous pollination, out-crossing rate, temporal and spatial distribution, SSR markers, genetic diversity, population structure

1. Introduction

Pollination relations occur among all existing forms of *Brassica napus* L. from different habitats; crops (mainly oilseed rape varieties), volunteers (grown from seed losses in previous years inside cultivated areas), and feral populations (appearing outside cultivation areas, mainly along the transportation infrastructure) [1, 2]. In the case of coexistence of different cropping systems which includes genetically modified (GM) oilseed rape production, introduction of transgenes in *B. napus* or related species is possible [3–7]. In nature, spontaneous inter-specific hybridization of *B. napus* is possible with sexually compatible species (relatives that have high pollination affinity with *B. napus*) from the Brassicaceae family. Villaseñor and Spinosa-Garcia [8] reported 7.3% of alien flowering plants in Mexico including 45 species and 25 genera from Brassicaceae family compared with 5.1% of its alien floras of the world determined by Pysek [9]. The relatives of *B. napus* are cultivated as field crops, but can also appear as weeds or wild outside cultivated areas (e.g., field edges, shelterbelts, road verges, slag heaps, embankments) [4, 6, 10]. Unpredicted persistence of all existing forms of *B. napus* in the agro-ecosystem is the most common consequence of preservation and self-recruitment of seeds originating from soil seed bank [11–15]. Because of its physical characteristics, the seed is very mobile and therefore disposed to spillage. Uncontrolled seed loss represents the potential for the appearance of volunteer and feral populations of *B. napus* inside and outside production areas; *B. napus* seed remains viable in the soil for several years [16, 17]. The population dynamics of these plants is dependent on the soil seed bank potential and on the complex interactive characteristics of the genotype, soil, and agro-climatic factors [18–23]. Pollen transfer is a primary source of gene flow and has direct influence on the level of genetic exchange within and among plants, depending on the landscape context within which it occurs [24, 25]. Non-native *B. napus* invasions and migrations are possible by vehicles, which act as vectors of long-distance dispersal [26, 27]. The spread of biological propagules, both pollen and seeds, plays a pivotal role in a number of fundamental ecological and evolutionary processes [28]. Dispersal is a process of central importance for the ecological and evolutionary dynamics of populations and communities, because of its diverse consequences for gene flow and demography [29]. The presence of undefined pollination in both natural and agricultural systems presents the potential for spontaneous intra- and inter-specific hybridization, reflected in the genetic structure and biodiversity of *B. napus*.

B. napus originated through spontaneous inter-specific hybridization (followed by polyploidization) between turnip rape (*B. rapa* L.; genome AA, 2n = 20) and cabbage (*B. oleracea* L.; genome CC, 2n = 18), resulting in an allotetraploid genome comprising the full chromosome complements of its two progenitors. Spontaneous hybridization between *B. rapa* and *B. oleracea* (from Europe and Asia) occurred due to contemporary cultivation of both species in a small geographic area in the Mediterranean region [30].

B. napus is a self-pollinated plant species with a variable out-crossing rate, influenced by genotype and environmental conditions. Due to the variable out-crossing rate, intra- and inter-specific gene flow may occur in nature [30–32]. Inside cultivation areas, the common rate of out-crossing is from 20 to 30% [23]. The out-crossing rate between different varieties with full fertility is up to 0.1% on the field-to-field scale, while in varieties with incorporated male sterility (bait plants; they produce no pollen on their own and represent the worst case scenario on the out-crossing rate), it is higher than 1% [23, 33]. Out-crossing potential is most prominent on field margins and starts diminishing after 10 m; however, pollination at greater distances is not excluded. This is more frequent in cases where there are no other flowering plants in the surroundings of the donor plant/cultivated crop. The out-crossing rate is significantly influenced by proportions between donor and recipient plants [23].

Different marker systems including short sequence repeat (SSR) markers are used for genetic characterization of agro-economically important plant species [10, 34–37]. To assess the molecular variation, genetic structure and gene flow potential among *B. napus* genome on a spatial and temporal scale, proved to be best suitable applying several molecular marker systems (RAPD, AFLP, SINE, ISSR, and SSR) [1, 6, 38–40]. There are also newly developed DNA marker types (e.g., SNP, KASP-SNP) and NGS (Next Generation Sequencing) based applications (e.g., GWS, GBS, RAD) [41–44] for genotyping and breeding purposes of *B. napus*.

Fragmented landscape and small-sized field structure reflect the heterogeneous growth conditions in several parts of Europe and world. The presence of ecological barriers like landscape structural elements (small woods, hedges, overgrown paths, and hills) and the influence of different agro-climatic conditions manage pollen and seed distribution [45]. Consequently, the persistence of *B. napus* plants originating from seed in soil seed banks enables gene flow potential on a spatial and temporal scale, reflecting in the crop quality, seed purity, and long-term biodiversity. Therefore, the aim of this study is to empirically estimate the out-crossing potential of *B. napus* gene transfer, under a fragmented landscape (10 statistical regions) in Slovenia and study the conservation of spontaneous gene flow into *B. napus* genome on a temporal level (4-year period). Through analysis of genetic diversity and calculation of population genetics parameters, implemented by advanced bioinformatics procedures, this study represents the important agronomical, biological, and ecological baselines. The presented results are provided on a DNA level, which is the most reliable way to determine changes in the genetic composition of *B. napus* genome on a spatial and temporal scale. Our goals were (a) to identify the distribution pattern and population dynamics of volunteers and feral populations along statistical regions in Slovenia; (b) to assess the global diversity of naturally appearing gene pool structure of *B. napus*; (c) to evaluate the genetic differentiation between volunteers and feral populations; (d) to obtain the spatial and temporal distribution of spontaneous pollination potential and estimation of gene flow conservation; (e) to find the empirically assigned out-crossing rate of *B. napus* under a fragmented landscape structure during a 4-year period of monitoring; (f) to observe that due to genetic diversity and population genetics parameters, ecologically, evolutionary, and agronomically oriented studies could be conducted at the DNA level using highly informative SSR markers.

2. Materials and methods

2.1. Study area

For the purpose of the study, we have selected macro-locations on a regional level—regions along Slovenia with high crop production share of *B. napus* (as oilseed rape) [2]. Therefore, from all statistical regions (12) of Slovenia, 10 were included in our research (Osrednjeslovenska-OSR,

Gorenjska-GOR, Jugovzhodna Slovenia-JVS, Notranjsko-kraška-NTK, Obalno-kraška-OBK, Podravska-POD, Pomurska-POM, Savinjska-SAV, Spodnjeposavska-SPS, and Zasavska-ZAS) (**Figure 1**). Inside those regions, we identified agrotopes (field edges, meadows, loess slopes, shelterbelts, field margins, field paths, etc.) and ruderal habitats (road verges, railway embankments, slag heaps, construction sites, rest areas by the roads, uncultivated areas, mounds, roundabouts, etc.) as main orientation points for field survey. Meanwhile, volunteer populations were sampled inside field margins as weedy plants in other cultivated crops.

2.2. Field survey

Field survey was conducted in a 4-year period from 2007 to 2010 every year during the flowering time of the biennial *B. napus* (third week of April and first week of May). We sampled five young leaves from each individual plant per population from each micro-location on an area of approx. 5m^2 including a minimum of five plants of *B. napus*. Sampled leaves were frozen (−20°C) and stored for DNA analysis.

2.3. DNA extraction

The leaf apex of each sample from the five young plants was bulked for DNA extraction with BioSprint 15 DNA Plant Kit (Qiagen) on a KingFisher (Thermo) isolation robot following the optimized method according to manufacturer's instructions.

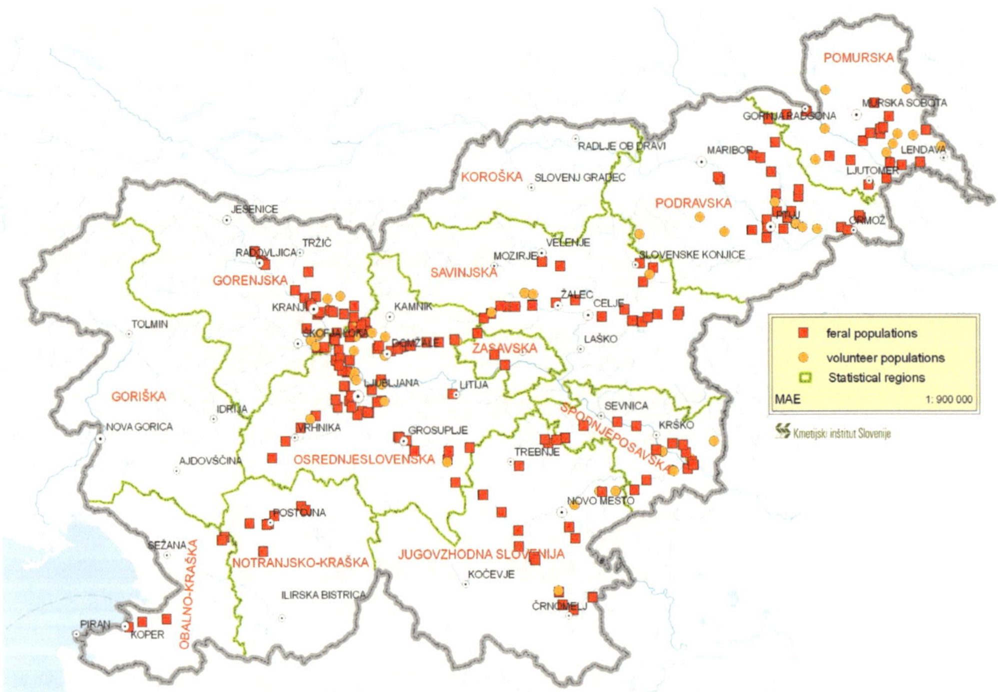

Figure 1. Sampling locations of feral and volunteer populations of *B. napus* in 2007–2010 along Slovenian statistical regions.

2.4. Genotyping procedure

A total of 45 nuclear SSR markers originating from different Brassicaceae family species, with various nucleotide repeat motives (listed in **Table 1**) were used. Thirty-seven SSR markers (with Na, Ol, Ni, Ra) were developed by Lowe et al. [46]; two SSR markers (with BRMS) were published by Suwabe et al. [47]; two SSR markers (with MR) were by Uzanova and Ecke [48]; one SSR marker (named BN83B1) was developed by Szewc-McFadden et al. [49]; and two SSR markers (with RES) were published by Wang et al. [50]. PCR reactions were performed on a final volume of 11.5 μl, containing 30 ng of genomic DNA and the following reagents with initial concentrations of: 10 x PCR buffer (Biotools), 10 mM of each dNTPs, 50 mM $MgCl_2$ (Biotools), 10 μM of each primer, 10 μM 5′ fluorescently labeled universal primer (6-FAM, NED, HEX), and 0. 5 U of Taq DNA polymerase (Biotools). The forward primer of each SSR was appended with 18 bp tail sequence 5′-TGTAAAACGACGGCCAGT-3′ (M13(−21) as described by Schuelke [51]. PCR analyses were performed on ATC 401 (Apollo Instrumentations) under the following "touch-down" conditions, dependent on each primer pair: 94°C for 4 min; 15 cycles at 94°C for 1 min; auto decrement temperature from 60 (62)°C at 0.7°C per cycle for 30 s; 72°C for 1 min, followed by 23 cycles at 94°C for 30 s; 53°C for 30 s; 72°C for 1 min; and final extension for 5 min at 72°C. Fragment analysis was performed on a 3130XL genetic analyzer (ABI); the allele lengths were determined by comparison to a size standard GeneScan-350 ROX (ABI) using GeneMapper 4.0 (ABI).

2.5. Data analysis

Parameters of genetic diversity among loci including ranges of allele lengths (Ra), numbers of alleles (n), frequencies of null alleles (No), and probability of identity (PI) were calculated using Identity v.1.0 [52]. MsToolkit [53] was used to evaluate expected heterozygosities (He), observed heterozygosities (Ho), and polymorphic information content (PIC). Locus-specific fixation indices and deviations of volunteer and feral populations from the Hardy–Weinberg equilibrium (HWE) were calculated using the GenAlEx v.6.4. [54]. Detecting the loci under selection was performed using Arlequin v.3.5.1.2 software [55] with 20,000 simulations. FSTAT v.2.9.3.2 [56] was used to determine allelic richness (R) as a measure of the number of alleles independent of sample size after 2000 permutations. The calculations of population statistics parameters at the spatial and temporal level including numbers of different alleles (Na), numbers of private alleles (Np), numbers of effective alleles (Ne), number of locally common alleles, fixation indices (F), population-specific expected heterozygosities (He), Shannon's information index (I), and pairwise Nei's genetic correlations were obtained using GenAlEx v.6.4 [54]. The out-crossing rate (t) was calculated from the fixation index using the equation $t = (1 - F) / (1 + F)$ described by He et al. [57]. Gene flow among volunteer and feral populations was estimated by calculating the effective number of migrants (m) using the private allele method of Slatkin [58], implemented by Genepop v.4.1 [59]; the corrected estimated value of Barton and Slatkin were reported [60]. Two common estimators of volunteer and feral population differentiation (Fst and Rst as standard parameters of genetic distance) are Fst, based on allele identity, and Rst, which incorporates the SSR-specific stepwise mutation model. Calculations of both estimations were performed using GenAlEx v.6.4 [54], where the estimation of RST was evaluated by AMOVA with 999 permutations. Pairwise genetic and geographic (log10 [lat, long]) uniformity between genotypes in the 4-year period, was established by 999 permutations with the Mantel test [61]. The mean within region pairwise values (r), according

Locus	Repeat motif	Ra[bp]	n	He	Ho	N_0	PI	PIC	F
Na12-A07	(GT/CA)$_{11}$	160–190	13	0.601	0.473	0.077	0.197	0.573	0.003
Na12-B05	(GA/CT)$_{18}$	135–221	27	0.862	0.767	0.034	0.030	0.845	0.005
Na12-C08	(GA/CT)$_{50}$	259–349	21	0.711	0.388	0.169	0.107	0.691	0.008
Na12-E05	(GT/CA)$_{10}$	102–176	21	0.730	0.866	−0.078	0.099	0.704	0.003
Na12-G05	(GA/CT)$_{50}$	144–254	22	0.876	0.749	0.069	0.027	0.858	0.005
Na14-E11	(GA/CT)$_{29}$	108–184	16	0.722	0.871	−0.077	0.117	0.678	0.001
Na14-G02	(GA/CT)$_{17}$	139–215	16	0.817	0.729	0.045	0.059	0.791	0.008
Ni3-G04b	(GA/CT)$_{18}$	99–171	20	0.690	0.747	−0.033	0.138	0.641	0.002
Ni4-D09	(GA/CT)$_{25}$	162–246	22	0.911	0.932	−0.008	0.016	0.899	0.002
Ni4-E08	(GA/CT)$_{47}$	105–195	11	0.422	0.436	−0.017	0.394	0.388	0.005
Na12-A08	(GA/CT)$_{28}$	137–205	17	0.778	0.415	0.203	0.066	0.753	0.003
Na12-E06a	(GA/CT)$_{23'}$	162–252	12	0.816	0.730	0.052	0.055	0.790	0.006
Na12-C06	(GA/CT)$_{37}$	153–285	19	0.895	0.702	0.095	0.213	0.880	0.002
Na10-A08	(GA/CT)$_{21}$	107–217	21	0.700	0.723	−0.012	0.118	0.677	0.002
Na14-H11	(GT/CA)$_{10}$	102–182	15	0.758	0.969	−0.120	0.091	0.725	0.005
BN83B1	(GA)$_{11}$ (AAG)$_{4}$	135–232	13	0.414	0.201	0.139	0.393	0.396	0.011
MR183	(TG)$_{11}$	80–116	12	0.743	0.938	−0.106	0.108	0.699	0.001
Ni4-G04	(GA/CT)$_{60}$	260–348	10	0.619	0.350	0.147	0.205	0.562	0.007
Ni4-H04	(GT/CA)$_{14}$	132–134	16	0.872	0.253	0.334	0.026	0.848	0.029
Ol10-D03	(GA/CT)$_{20}$	106–190	21	0.793	0.938	−0.089	0.067	0.767	0.003
Ol11-D12	(GA/CT)$_{52}$	111–209	32	0.931	0.685	0.145	0.009	0.920	0.007
Ol11-G11	(GGC/CCG)$_{5}$	99–197	15	0.831	0.959	−0.065	0.051	0.806	0.004
Ol11-H02	(AAT/AAG)$_{18}$	128–218	12	0.802	0.713	0.047	0.070	0.772	0.003
Ol12-A04	(GA/CT)$_{17}$	120–202	15	0.449	0.410	0.023	0.328	0.428	0.002
Ol12-B05	(GA/CT)$_{36}$	122–244	20	0.516	0.405	0.069	0.256	0.493	0.004
Ol12-D05	(GA/CT)$_{32}$	101–193	17	0.770	0.665	0.048	0.068	0.745	0.003
Ol12-D09	(GGC/CCG)$_{4}$	103–193	11	0.703	0.875	−0.095	0.118	0.653	0.007
Ol12-E03	(GGC/CCG)$_{9}$	94–257	13	0.854	0.921	−0.045	0.039	0.832	0.001
Ol12-F11	(GT/CA)$_{14}$	124–254	17	0.707	0.660	0.023	0.130	0.678	0.016
Ol13-E08	(GA/CT)$_{11}$	126–232	17	0.729	0.770	−0.043	0.118	0.684	0.002
Ra2-A01	(GA/CT)$_{19}$	98–144	12	0.671	0.910	−0.149	0.171	0.611	0.001
Ra2-A10	(GT/CA)$_{107}$	170–296	13	0.648	0.313	0.195	0.177	0.608	0.007
Ra2-E03	(GA/CT)$_{18}$	187–319	19	0.589	0.334	0.165	0.226	0.555	0.010
Ra2-E04	(GA/CT)$_{19}$	96–218	18	0.657	0.925	−0.155	0.174	0.593	0.002
Ra2-E12	(GA/CT)$_{32}$	115–281	24	0.782	0.769	0.018	0.069	0.757	0.002

Locus	Repeat motif	Ra[bp]	n	He	Ho	N_0	PI	PIC	F
Ra2-F11	$(GA/CT)_{34}$	151–307	29	0.797	0.929	−0.068	0.065	0.768	0.003
Ra2-G09	$(GA/CT)_{19}$	168–266	21	0.740	0.461	0.159	0.096	0.717	0.007
Ra3-E05	$(GT/CA)_{65}$	183–285	11	0.656	0.735	−0.038	0.165	0.607	0.003
Ra3-H10	$(GA/CT)_{23}$	122–202	13	0.779	0.823	−0.025	0.072	0.760	0.006
BRMS-036	$(CA)_{10}(GA)_4$	100–178	15	0.813	0.976	−0.082	0.055	0.786	0.001
BRMS-050	$(AAT)_4(TC)_{19}(TTC)_3$	143–215	14	0.361	0.292	0.047	0.473	0.345	0.013
MR187	$(AG)_{23}(AGG)_5$	101–189	18	0.600	0.450	0.103	0.175	0.579	0.001
RES1	$(CCT)_5$	104–199	16	0.812	0.912	−0.058	0.064	0.782	0.002
RES6	$(ATG)_7$	148–223	10	0.373	0.244	0.088	0.426	0.352	0.003
BN6A2	$(GATT)_4$	93–133	9	0.596	0.415	0.116	0.191	0.556	0.003
Total			**756**				**2.480×10^{-46}**		
Mean			**16.8**	**0.709**	**0.661**	**0.028**		**0.679**	**0.005**

*Range of allele lengths (Ra), number of alleles (n), expected heterozygosity (He), observed heterozygosity (Ho), estimated frequency of null alleles (No), probability of identity (PI), polymorphic information content (PIC), and fixation index (F).

Table 1. Parameters of genetic diversity within volunteer and feral populations among loci*.

to geographic and genetic distance, was calculated by 999 permutations and 1000 bootstraps using GenAlEx v.6.4 [54]. To assess the genetic structure of volunteer and feral populations, a Bayesian method was used. This analysis was performed using the model-based software Structure v.2.3.3 [62] that infers the number of genetic groups K present in a sample by comparing the posterior probability for different numbers of putative populations specified by the user and assigning individuals, giving a percentage of membership (Q value), for these clusters. The admixture model with 100,000 MCMC (Markov chain Monte Carlo) repetitions and 10,000 burn-in periods were used. Eleven independent runs were performed without prior information on groups assuming correlated allele frequencies. Temporal changes of genetic structure among volunteer and feral populations were estimated in PCoA (principal coordinate analysis) via covariance matrix with data standardization using GenAlEx v.6.4. [54].

3. Results

3.1. The dataset

In the 4-year period, 261 samples were collected in total—66 samples of volunteer populations and 195 samples of feral populations within 10 statistical regions in Slovenia (**Figure 1**).

3.2. Evaluation of genetic diversity

Genotypic results for 45 analyzed loci are summarized in **Table 1**. All loci were 100% polymorphic in both volunteer and feral populations. The selected set of SSR markers is highly applicable for genetic differentiation analysis within *B. napus* genome, suggesting high mean PIC value (0.679) and low total PI value (2.480×10^{-46}) (**Table 1**). The most informative locus with the highest PIC value was Ni4-D09, which originated from *B. nigra* genome (**Table 1**). Global genetic diversity (mean He value, **Table 1**) between all naturally present volunteer and feral populations in Slovenia is 0.709. Positive and low mean N_0 value (**Table 1**) suggests that there was negligible mutation activity within the included SSR regions in *B. napus* genome, during the 4-year period.

According to the exact HWE test, both volunteer and feral populations do not meet HWE conditions ($P < 0.05$) for any of the 45 loci, which is confirmed by the mean positive value of F (0.005) (**Table 1**), indicating spontaneous random mating and inbreeding potential. These findings reflect the characteristics of natural populations during the 4-year monitoring of non-cultivated *B. napus* populations. Significant changes ($P < 0.05$) in genetic structure of all included genotypes at each locus were detected for loci Ra3-H10 and NA10-A08; it is assumed that the level of gene flow for those loci was influenced by microevolution and natural selection. The calculated values of different alleles (Na = 12.40), private alleles (Np = 1.13), and fixation index (F = 0.072) within volunteer populations were lower compared to feral populations, where Na was 15.67, Np reached 4.40, and F was 0.074. Naturally occurring out-crossing rate among feral populations during the 4-year period on the national level is 13.71%; the global out-crossing rate among volunteer populations is lower (13.47%). These comparisons indicate the favorable introduction and conservation of new alleles via spontaneous gene flow in nature in self-recruited generations of feral populations.

The MCMC structure of 45 SSRs showed moderate genetic structure. When Evanno's [63] ad hoc estimator of the real number of clusters was used, it indicated modes at K = 3 (**Figure 2**). The average genetic distances between genotypes in the first cluster is 0.794 (Fst = 0.062), following 0.627 (Fst = 0.169) in the second cluster and 0.646 (Fst = 0.092) in the third genetic cluster.

3.3. Regional-spatial assessment of gene flow in fragmented field landscapes

Genetic diversity and allelic structure of volunteer and feral populations along statistical regions are presented in **Figure 3** and **Table 2**. According to the highest values of expected heterozygosity (He) and Shannon's information index (I), the most genetically diverse genotypes are from JVS (He = 0.731; I = 1.779), SAV (He = 0.726; I = 1.729), OSR (He = 0.688; I = 1.627), and POM (He = 0.662; I = 1.482) regions (**Figure 3**). The highest number of private alleles, Np = 0.867, was detected among genotypes from OSR (**Figure 3**); the out-crossing rate inside this region reached 10.45%. The highest out-crossing rate was calculated within SAV (*t* = 18.75%) and

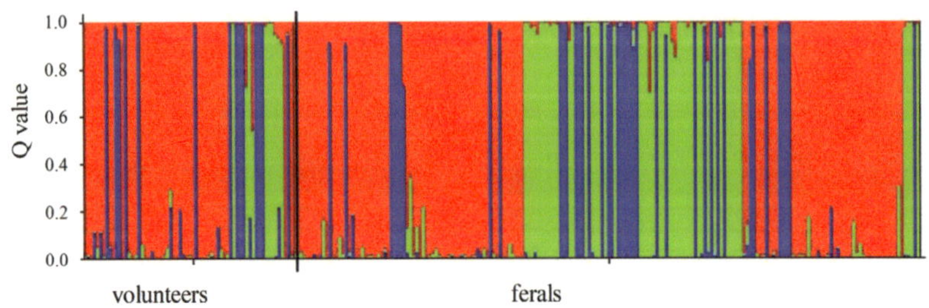

Figure 2. Genetic structure of volunteer and feral populations, according to three genetic clusters.

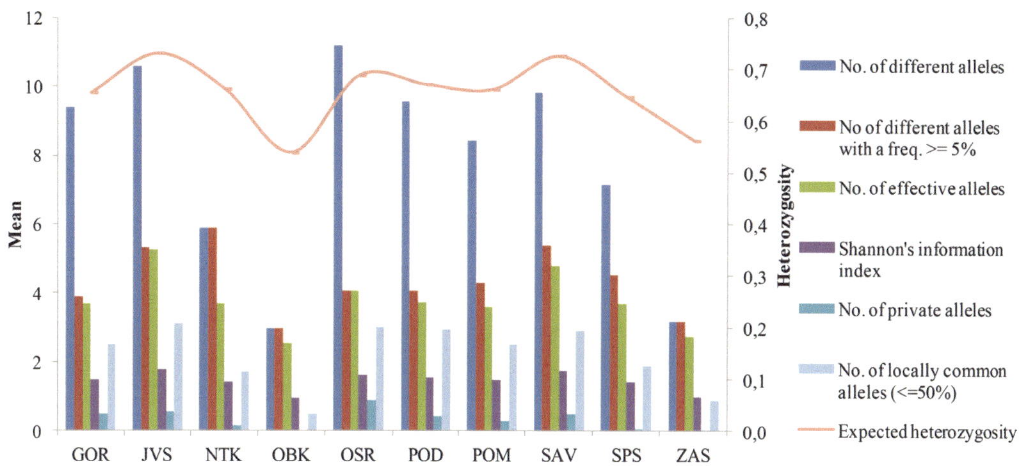

Figure 3. Genetic patterns according to spatial distribution of volunteer and feral populations.

JVS (t = 18.31%) regions. The differences between the highest Np and low t values in the OSR region indicate the favorable potential of gene flow conservation in feral and volunteer populations; this is in contrast with the JVS and SAV regions, where the level of spontaneous gene flow was high, but conservation into naturally occurred populations, was low.

The estimation of R_{ST} (using stepwise mutation model) using AMOVA showed 4% molecular variability among statistical regions. High genetic relatedness between genotypes from different

	GOR	JVS	NTK	OBK	OSR	POD	POM	SAV	SPS	ZAS
GOR	*	0.032	0.020	0.076	0.006	0.010	0.010	0.017	0.012	0.070
JVS	0.857	*	0.034	0.096	0.026	0.027	0.030	0.015	0.038	0.066
NTK	0.919	0.850	*	0.093	0.019	0.019	0.022	0.020	0.022	0.072
OBK	0.820	0.724	0.761	*	0.073	0.079	0.077	0.085	0.088	0.122
OSR	0.977	0.874	0.921	0.826	*	0.009	0.009	0.012	0.013	0.067
POD	0.958	0.874	0.921	0.801	0.963	*	0.010	0.015	0.016	0.063
POM	0.963	0.865	0.911	0.813	0.963	0.955	*	0.014	0.017	0.067
SAV	0.929	0.923	0.915	0.772	0.941	0.934	0.940	*	0.021	0.061
SPS	0.957	0.842	0.913	0.788	0.951	0.937	0.936	0.919	*	0.068
ZAS	0.770	0.763	0.764	0.711	0.774	0.789	0.774	0.785	0.778	*

*Upper (U) and lower (L) confidence limits bound the 95% confidence interval about the null hypothesis of "No difference" across the regions as determined by permutation. The lowest mean r value was calculated across POD region (63.3%), where r was outside U and L limits reflecting the highest genetic and geographic difference of included genotypes along this region.

Table 2. Values of pairwise comparisons of feral and volunteer populations according to statistical regions, Nei's genetic identity (under diagonal) and F_{ST} values (above diagonal).

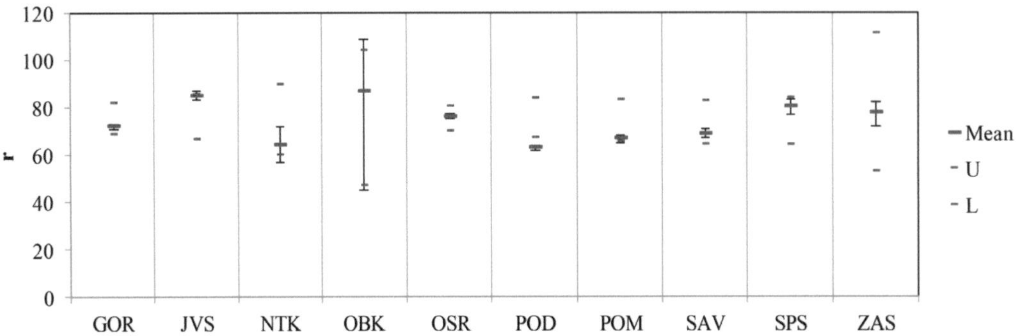

Figure 4. Mean within region pairwise values (r), according to geographic and genetic distance.

regions was also confirmed with pairwise comparisons between genotypes from different geographical areas, based on Nei's genetic identity and F_{ST} values (**Table 2**). The highest pairwise genetic correlation was calculated between genotypes from the OSR and GOR regions (0.977), which corresponds to the lowest F_{ST} values, based on allele frequencies between these two geographic areas (F_{ST} = 0.006) (**Table 2**). These two regions are geographically neighboring areas (**Figure 1**).

According to the results from **Table 2**, the included genotypes are relatively homogenously dispersed along all geographic areas and no grouping of genetically similar genotypes within statistical regions was observed. This finding was confirmed by a global Mantel test, which compares the genetic and geographic distance matrix of all 261 genotypes. The Mantel correlation coefficient of genetic and spatial relatedness between genotypes was low, but positive (rxy = 0.044, P = 0.01), due to minor spatial linkage on the basis of genetic structure. The summary of the mean within region pairwise values, based on genetic and geographic distance, is presented in **Figure 4**.

3.4. Temporal distribution of landscape gene flow and conservation of genetic variation

Temporal distribution of genetic variation, according to 100% polymorphic loci during the 4-year monitoring is presented in **Table 3**. Increasing values of Np, m, and molecular variance for every successive year, signify the gene flow potential, distribution, and conservation of new alleles into *B. napus* genome in a relatively short period. However, for allelic richness, the highest contribution was determined in 2010 (see **Table 3**).

According to PCoA results, there is a decreasing pattern of genetic linkages between all genotypes from 2007 to 2010 (**Figure 5**). This genetic differentiation reflects the spontaneous gene flow through the 4-year period in the surveyed agro-ecosystem.

4. Discussion

According to the 4-year field monitoring, volunteer/feral populations appeared within statistical regions, where *B. napus* have been widely cultivated as oilseed rape (OSR, 56; GOR,

45; POD, 36; JVS, 32; POM and SAV, 29). The actual regional cultivation of *B. napus* in 2009 was reported by Pipan et al. [2], where the highest proportion of oilseed rape production was inscribed along POM and POD regions. There was no volunteer or feral population found inside Goriška and Koroška region. Distribution of volunteer and feral populations (**Figure 1**) represents the highly-developed *B. napus* persistence under the Slovenian fragmented landscape structure, according to soil seed bank potential as a consequence of seed movements. The regional pattern of *B. napus* presence indicates that volunteer or feral populations most commonly originate from seed losses. Zhu et al. [17] report that seed losses during harvest could be limited to 0.7–1.1% of total seed production under Chinese farming systems. Consequently, uncultivated forms of *B. napus* colonize mostly pioneer habitats, such as waste sites, cultivated grounds, rubble tips, arable fields, riverbanks, road sides, and tracks [6, 64].

In this study, spatial and temporal determination of genetic changes on 45 loci inside the *B. napus* genome was proven to be useful and informative—there was low probability of identity value (PI = 2.480×10^{-46}) and high polymorphic content value (PIC = 0.679) (see **Table 1**) among single species. These values also reflect the equal distribution of alleles among volunteer and feral genotypes. SSR markers are suitable to identify varieties of *B. napus* (e.g., [6, 39, 65]). A high level of genetic differentiation within the same species was obtained in our study. The composed structure of some SSR repeat motives, which originated from *Brassica sp.* (BN83B1, PIC = 0.396; BRMS-050, PIC = 0.345), could have a negative effect on the information content (**Table 1**). We would like to emphasize the highly distinctive loci RES1 (PI = 0.782, **Table 1**) developed from the sexually compatible relative of *B. napus*, *Raphanussativus* [50]. This study confirmed the finding reported by Elling et al. [38], Hasan et al. [39], Suwabe et al. [47], and Bond et al. [66] that SSR markers originating from related *Brassica* species are highly applicable in investigations of *B. napus* gene pool.

Variable out-crossing rate, being a biological characteristic of *B. napus*, is 5–47% [30]. Likewise, empirically determined out-crossing rate in Slovenia was 13.6% and represents the spontaneous gene flow potential of *B. napus* under a fragmented landscape structure during a 4-year period. Moreover, the ability for introgression and conservation of spontaneous gene flow into *B. napus* genome through (self-recruited) generations in nature is possible. According to the increasing pattern of Np and m values in each following year during the 4-year period (**Table 3**), proves that genetic changes within volunteer/feral populations are reflected temporally. This finding is confirmed by PCoA distribution, where genetic relatedness between genotypes decreased (**Figure 5**) and the proportion of molecular variance during the 4-year period increased (**Table 3**). Additionally, genetic diversity within feral populations was higher, compared to volunteers due to uncontrolled pollination and introduction of new genes into feral populations. Pascher et al. [6] reported that feral populations shared less than 50% of the SSR alleles among 8 loci, compared to commercial varieties, which were cultivated in the previous year along the same region. Our results showed that alleles from both volunteer and feral populations were distributed in three genetic clusters (**Figure 2**) with relatively similar level of diversity. Considering this, we assume that high proportion of spatially and temporary distributed agro-biodiversity of *B. napus* gene pool was observed (global He = 0.709, F = 0.005; **Table 1**). Temporal determination among volunteers and feral populations was described by R, a measure of independent quantitative comparison of genetic diversity between all years. Overall, the most genetically diverse genotypes were

Parameter of population diversity and genetics	Ecological interpretation	2007	2008	2009	2010
Ne	Allelic diversity	4.01	3.80	3.64	4.17
Np	Estimation of spontaneous gene flow conservation into naturally appearing populations	0.58	0.93	0.98	1.64
F	Estimated level of spontaneous gene flow	0.03	0.01	0.07	0.05
t (%)	Actual gene flow potential	5.74	2.81	13.27	12.52
Molecular variance (%)	Conservation of naturally occurring spontaneous gene flow	1.64	1.78	2.77	6.1
m	Level of gene flow	2.16	3.36	4.41	5.47
R	Basic genetic diversity parameter; allelic richness	3.41	1.67	3.23	5.64

Table 3. Ecologically important parameters of population genetics for genetic diversity distribution in 4-year sampling period.

determined in 2010, additionally confirmed with the highest Ne value (**Table 3**), indicating the ability and introduction of new alleles through spontaneous pollination of *B. napus* in nature.

Our study suggests that there is no specific distribution of genetically similar genotypes present within the same statistical region. Conversely, the proportion of shared molecular variability of volunteers/feral populations between regions is high (96%). These large-scale genetic similarities could be caused by common ancestry from commercial varieties of *B. napus*

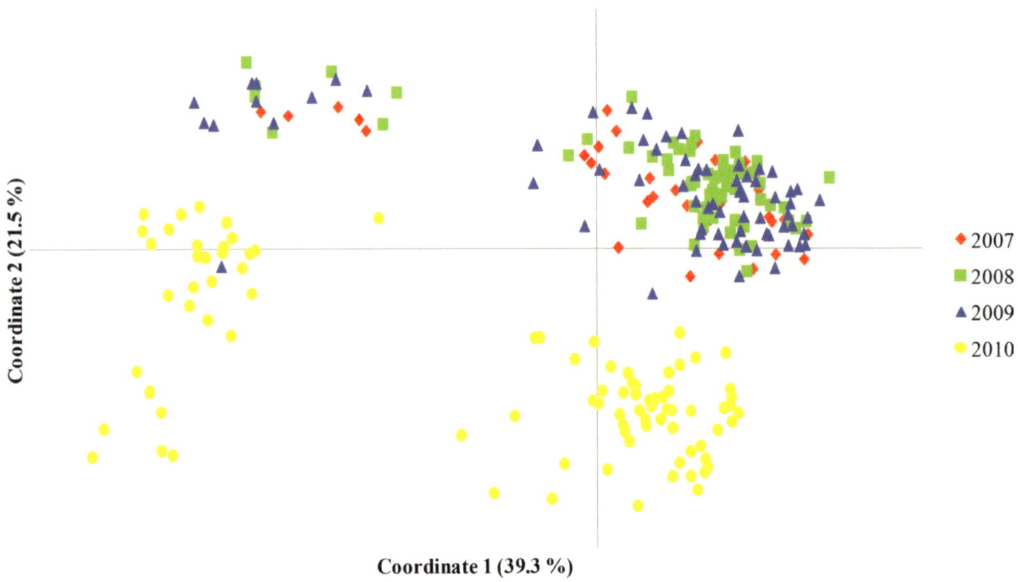

Figure 5. PCoA temporal distribution of genotypes.

(oilseed rape), which were cultivated in the observed statistical regions. Pasher et al. [6] observed that genetic similarities among feral populations could be caused by selection favoring or eliminating certain alleles of loci linked to the markers, or by pollination and hybridization with sexually compatible relatives. However, Mantel correlation coefficient between genetic and geographic distance matrix assigned a low level of spatially and genetically related distribution among genotypes. The highest spatially distributed genetic diversity was observed in the JVS and SAV regions (He >0.700; **Figure 3**); the highest numbers of locally common alleles (< 50%) with a frequency > 5% (**Figure 3**) were detected along the JVS and OSR regions. Most likely, the highest potential for gene flow conservation into natural *B. napus* populations (highest Np values) was determined within the OSR region (**Figure 3**) due to favorable agro-climatic and geographic conditions. The most genetically heterogeneous genotypes, according to their spatial position, were formed along the POD region (**Figure 3**).

5. Conclusions

Distribution of volunteer and feral populations represents the highly developed *B. napus* persistence under the Slovenian fragmented landscape structure, according to soil seed bank potential as a consequence of seed movements. The regional pattern of *B. napus* presence indicates that volunteer/feral populations most commonly originate from seed losses. In this study, spatial and temporal determination of genetic changes on 45 loci within *B. napus* genome was proven to be useful and informative. Empirically determined out-crossing rate in Slovenia was 13.6% and represents the spontaneous gene flow potential of *B. napus*, under a fragmented landscape structure during a 4-year period. This calculation reflects that the actual large-scale situation is an important basis for ecological, agronomical, and ecological evaluation of spontaneous pollination potential of *B. napus* in this agro-ecosystem. Moreover, the ability of introgression and conservation of spontaneous gene flow into the *B. napus* genome through (self-recruited) generations in nature is possible. Our study suggests that there is no specific distribution of genetically similar genotypes present within the same statistical region.

Our empirically obtained results show the existing potential of large-scale spontaneous pollination and gene flow conservation into the *B. napus* gene pool in a short time period under a fragmented landscape structure. Genetic diversity of naturally present *B. napus* plants and spatially and temporally determined conservation of genetic variation, is proven to be successfully assessed using SSR markers, due to biologically, agronomically, evolutionary, and ecologically important parameters.

Acknowledgements

The authors acknowledge the financial support from the Slovenian Research Agency (research core funding No. (Agrobiodiversity P4-0072 and Young researcher grant: B. Pipan, contract number 1000-07-310099)). We are also grateful to MatejKnapič for spatial visualization of sampling locations.

Author details

Vladimir Meglič* and Barbara Pipan

*Address all correspondence to: vladimir.meglic@kis.si

Crop Science Department, Agricultural Institute of Slovenia, Ljubljana, Slovenia

References

[1] Pascher K, Narendja F, Rau D. Feral oilseed rape-investigations on its potential hybridisation. Final Report in Commission of the Federal Ministry of Health and Women. Vienna, Austria: Federal Ministry of Health and Women; 2006

[2] Pipan B, Šuštar-Vozlič J, Meglič V. Cultivation, varietal structure and possibilities for cross-pollination of *Brassica napus* L. in Slovenia. ActaAgiculturea Slovenica. 2011;**97**: 247-258

[3] Devaux C, Klein EK, Lavigne C, Sausse C, Messean A. Environmental and landscape effects on cross-pollination rates observed at long distance among French oilseed rape *Brassica napus* commercial fields. Journal of Applied Ecology. 2008;**45**:803-812

[4] Eastham K, Sweet J. Genetically modified organisms (GMOs): The significance of gene flow through pollen transfer. Environmental Issue Report. 2002;**28**:15-26

[5] Garnier A, Lecomte J. Using a spatial and stage-structured invasion model to assess the spread of feral populations of transgenic oilseed rape. Ecological Modelling. 2006;**194**:141-149

[6] Pascher K, Macalka S, Rau D, Gollman G, Reiner H, Glössl J, Grabherr G. Molecular differentiation of commercial varieties and feral populations of oilseed rape (*Brassica napus* L.). BMC Evolutinary Biology. 2010;**10**:63. DOI: 10.1186/1471-2148-10-63

[7] Liu Y, Wei W, Ma K, Li J, Liang Y, Darmency H. Consequences of gene flow between oilseed rape (*Brassica napus*) and its relatives. Plant Science. 2013;**211**:42-51

[8] Villaseñor JL, Espinosa-Garcia FJ. The alien flowering plants of Mexico. Diversity and Distributions. 2004;**10**:113-123

[9] Pysek P. Is there a taxonomic pattern to plant invasions? Oikos. 1998;**82**:282-294

[10] Pipan B, Šuštar-Vozlič J, Meglič V. Genetic differentiation among sexually compatible relatives of *Brassica napus* L. Genetika. 2013;**45**:309-327

[11] Colbach N, Granger S, Mézière D. Using a sensitivity analysis of a weed dynamics model to develop sustainable cropping systems. II. Long-term effect of past crops and management techniques on weed infestation. The Journal of Agricultural Science. 2013;**151**:247-267

[12] Debeljak M, Squire G, Demšar D, Young MW, Džeroski S. Relations between the oilseed rape volunteer seed bank, and soil factors, weed functional groups and geographical location in the UK. Ecological Modelling. 2008;**212**:138-146

[13] Neubert MG, Caswell H. Demography and dispersal: Calculation and sensitivity analysis of invasion speed for structured populations. Ecology. 2000;**81**:1613-1628

[14] Pipan B, ŠuštarVozlič J, Meglič V. Preservation of *Brassica napus* L. seed in soil seed bank. Acta Agriculturae Slovenica. 2013;**101**:277-285

[15] Stump WL, Westra P. The seedbank dynamics of feral rye (*Secalecereale*). Weed Technology. 2000;**14**:7-14

[16] Pessel FD, Lecomte J, Emeriau V, Krouti M, Messean A, Gouyon PH. Persistence of oilseed rape (*Brassica napus* L.) outside of cultivated fields. Theoretical Applied Genetics. 2001;**102**:841-846

[17] Zhu YM, Li YD, Colbach N, Ma KP, Wei W, Mi XC. Seed losses at harvest and seed persistence of oilseed rape (*Brassica napus*) in different cultural conditions in Chinese farming systems. Weed Research. 2012;**52**:317-326

[18] Grappin P, Bouinot D, Sotta B, Miginiac E, Jullien M. Control of seed dormancy in *Nicotiana plumbaginifolia*: Post-imbibition abscisic acid synthesis imposes dormancy maintenance. Planta. 2000;**210**:279-285

[19] Gruber S, Bühler A, Möhring J, Claupein W. Sleepers in the soil-vertical distribution by tillage and long-term survival of oilseed rape seeds compared with plastic pellets. European Journal of Agronomy. 2010;**33**:81-88

[20] López-Granados F, Lutman PJW. Effect of environmental conditions on the dormancy and germination of volunteer oilseed rape seed (*Brassica napus*). Weed Science. 1998;**46**:419-423

[21] Momoh EJJ, Zhou WJ, Kristiansson B. Variation in the development of secondary seed dormancy in oilseed rape genotypes under conditions of stress. Weed Research. 2002;**42**:446-455

[22] Probert RJ. The role of temperature in germination ecophysiology. In: Fenner M, editor. Seeds: The Ecology of Regeneration in Plant Communities. 2nd ed. Wallingford: CAB International; 2000. pp. 285-325

[23] Squire GR, Begg GS, Askew M. The Potential for Oilseed Rape Feral (volunteer) Weeds to Cause Impurities in Later Oilseed Rape Crops. London, UK: Department of Environment, Food and Rural Affairs; 2003

[24] Rader R, Edwards W, Wetscott DA, Cunningham SA, Howlett BG. Pollen transport differs among bees and flies in a human-modified landscape. Diversity and Distributions. 2011;**17**:519-529

[25] Ottewell KM, Donnellana SC, Lowe AJ, Paton DC. Predicting reproductive success of insect-versus birdpollinated scattered trees in agricultural landscapes. Biological Conservation. 2009;**142**:888-898

[26] Von der Lippe M, Kowarik I. Do cities export biodiversity? Traffic as dispersal vector across urban-rural gradients. Diversity and Distributions. 2008;**14**:18-25

[27] Taylor K, Brummer T, Taper ML, Wing A, Rew LJ. Human-mediated long distance dispersal: An empirical evaluation of seed dispersal by vehicles. Diversity and Distributions. 2012;**18**:942-951

[28] Savage D, Barbetti MJ, MacLeod WJ, Salam MU, Renton M. Timing of propagule release significantly alters the deposition area of resulting aerial dispersal. Diversity and Distributions. 2010;**16**:288-299

[29] Saastamoinen M, Bocedi G, Cote J, et al. Genetics of dispersal. Biological Reviews. 2017;**93**:574-599. DOI: 10.1111/brv.12356

[30] Friedt W, Snowdon R. Oilseed rape. Oil crops. In: Vollman J, Rajcan I, editors. Handbook of Plant Breeding 4. Giessen: Springer Science+Business Media; 2009. pp. 91-126

[31] Snowdon R, Lühs W, Friedt W. Genome mapping and molecular breeding in plants. In: Kole C, editor. Oilseeds. 2nd ed. Berlin: Springer-Verlag; 2007. pp. 55-114

[32] Treu R.,Emberlin J. Pollen Dispersal of the Crops Maize (*Zea mays*), Oilseed Rape (*Brassica napus*), Potatoes (*Solanum tuberosum*), Sugar Beet (*Beta vulgaris*) and Wheat (*Triticum aestivum*). 2000. Bristol, UK: Soil Association, University College

[33] Ramsay G, Thompson C, Squire G. Quantifying Landscape-Scale Gene Flow in Oilseed Rape. London, UK: Department for Environment, Food and Rural Affairs; 2003

[34] Rusjan D, Pelengić R, Pipan B, Or E, Javornik B, Štajner N. Israeli germplasm: Phenotyping and genotyping of native grapevines (*Vitisvinifera* L.). Vitis. 2015;**54**:87-89

[35] Pipan B, Žnidarčič D, Meglič V. Evaluation of genetic diversity of sweet potato [*Ipomoea batatas* (L.) lam.] on different ploidy levels applying two capillary platforms. Journal of Horticultural Science and Biotechnology. 2016;**92**:192-198

[36] Maras M, Pipan B, Šuštar-Vozlič J, Todorović V, Đurić G, Vasić M, Kratovalieva S, Ibusoska A, Agić R, Matotan Z, Čupić T, Meglič V. Examination of genetic diversity of common bean from the western Balkans. Journal of the American Society for Horticultural Science. 2015;**140**:208-316

[37] Žnidarčič D, Vučajnik F, Ilin ŽM, Pipan B, Meglič V, Sinkovič L. The Influence of Different Substrates on the Growth, Yield and Quality of Slovenian Sweetpotato Cultivars under Greenhouse Conditions. Rijeka: InTech; 2018. forthcoming

[38] Elling B, Neuffer B, Bleeker W. Sources of genetic diversity in feral oilseed rape (*Brassica napus*) populations. Basic and Applied Ecology. 2009;**10**:544-553

[39] Hasan M, Seyis F, Badani AG, Pons-Kühnemann J, Friedt W, Lühs W, Snowdon RJ. Analysis of genetic diversity in the *Brassica napus* L. gene pool using SSR markers. Genetic Resources and Crop Evolution. 2006;**53**:793-802

[40] Hasan M, Friedt W, Pons-Kühnemann J, Freitag NM, Link K, Snowdon RJ. Association of gene-linked SSR markers to seed glucosinolate content in oilseed rape (*Brassica napus* ssp. *napus*). Theoretical Applied Genetics. 2008;**116**:1035-1049

[41] Clarke WE et al. A high-density SNP genotyping array for *Brassica napus* and its ancestral diploid species based on optimised selection of single-locus markers in the allotetraploid genome. Theoretical Applied Genetics. 2016;**129**:1887-1899

[42] Schmutzer T et al. Species-wide genome sequence and nucleotide polymorphisms from the model allopolyploid plant *Brassica napus*. Scientific Data. 2015;**2**:150072

[43] Lees CJ, Li G, Duncan RW. Characterization of *Brassica napus* L. genotypes utilizing sequence-related amplified polymorphism and genotyping by sequencing in association with cluster analysis. Molecular Breeding. 2016;**36**:155

[44] Bus A, Hecht J, Huettel B, Reinhardt R, Stich B. High-throughput polymorphism detection and genotyping in Brassica napus using next-generation RAD sequencing. BMC Genomics. 2012;**13**:281

[45] Pipan B. Genetska raznolikost navadne ogrščice (*Brassica napus* L.) in njenih spolno kompatibilnih sorodnikov v sloevnskem pridelovalnem prostoru [Doctoral thesis]. Ljubljana: Univerza v Ljubljani; 2013

[46] Lowe J, Moule C, Trick M, Edwards KJ. Efficient large-scale development of microsatellites for marker and mapping applications in *Brassica* crop species. Theoretical Applied Genetics. 2004;**108**:1103-1112

[47] Suwabe K, Iketani H, Nunome T, Kage T. Isolation and characterization of microsatellites in B. rapa. Theoretical Applied Genetics. 2002;**104**:1092-1098

[48] Uzanova MI, Ecke W. Abundance, polymorphism and genetic mapping of microsatellites in oilseed rape (*B. napus* L.). Plant Breeding. 1999;**118**:323-236

[49] Szewc-mcfadden K, Kresovich S, Bliek SM, Mitchell SE, Mcferson JR. Identification of polymorphic, conserved simple sequence repeats (SSRs) in cultivated Brassica species. Theoretical Applied Genetics. 1996;**93**:534-538

[50] Wang N, Hu J, Ohsawa R, Ohta M, Fujimura T. Identification and characterization of microsatellite markers derived from expressed sequence tags (ESTs) of radish (*Raphanus satvius* L.). Molecular Ecology Notes. 2007;**7**:503-506

[51] Schuelke M. An economic method for the fluorescent labelling of PCR fragments. Nature Biotechnology. 2000;**18**:233-234

[52] Wagner HW, Sefc KM. Identity 1.0. Vienna, Austria: Centre for Applied Genetics, University of Agricultural Sciences; 1999

[53] Park S. Microsatellite Toolkit. Dublin, Ireland: Department of Genetics, Trinity College; 2001

[54] Peakall R, Smouse PE. GenAlEx 6: Genetic analysis in Excel. Population genetic software for teaching and research. Molecular Ecology Notes. 2006;**6**:288-295

[55] Excoffier L, Lischer H. Arlequin suite ver 3.5: A new series of programs to perform population genetics analyses under Linux and Windows. Molecular Ecology Resources. 2010;**10**:564-567

[56] Goudet J. FSTAT: A Program to Estimate and Test Gene Diversities and Fixation Indices. Version 2.9.3.2. Lausanne, Switzerland: Institute of Ecology and Evolution, University of Lausanne; 2002

[57] He S, Wang Y, Volis S, Li D, Yi T. Genetic divrsity and population structure: Implications for conservation of wild soybean (Glycine sojaSieb. EtZucc) based on nuclear and chloroplast microsatellite variation. International Journal of Molecular Sciences. 2012;**13**:12608-12628

[58] Slatkin M. Gene flow in natural populations. Annual Review of Ecology and Systematics. 1985;**16**:393-430

[59] Rousset F. Genepop 4.1.0: A complete reimplementation of the Genepop software for Windows and Linux. Molecular Ecology Resources. 2008;**8**:103-106

[60] Barton NH, Slatkin M. A quasi-equilibrium theory of the distribution of rare alleles in a subdivided population. Heredity. 1986;**56**:409-416

[61] Mantel N. The detection of disease clustering and a generalized regression approach. Cancer Research. 1967;**27**:209-220

[62] Pritchard JK, Wen X, Falush D. Documentation for STRUCTURE Software: Version 2.3. USA: Department of Human Genetics, University of Chicago & Department of Statistics, University of Oxford; 2009

[63] Evanno G, Regnaut S, Goudet J. Detecting the number of clusters of individuals using the software STRUCTURE: A simulation study. Molecular Ecology. 2005;**14**:2611-2620

[64] Pivard S, Adamczyk K, Lecomte J, Lavigne C, Bouvier A, Deville A, Gouyon PH, Huet S. Where do the feral oilseed rape populations come from? A large-scale study of their possible origin in a farmland area. Journal of Applied Ecology. 2008;**45**:476-485

[65] Devaux C, Lavigne C, Falentin-Guyomarc'h H, Vautrin S, Lecomte J, Klein EK. High diversity of oilseed rape pollen clouds over an agro-ecosystem indicated long distance dispersal. Molecular Ecology. 2005;**14**:2269-2280

[66] Bond JM, Mogg RJ, Squire GR, Johnstone C. Microsatellite amplification in *Brassica napus* cultivars: Cultivar variability and relationship to a long-term feral population. Euphytica. 2004;**139**:173-178

Chapter 4

Pale-Green Kohlrabi, a Versatile *Brassica* Vegetable

Ana-Alexandra Sorescu, Alexandrina Nuta and
Rodica-Mariana Ion

Additional information is available at the end of the chapter

http://dx.doi.org/10.5772/intechopen.76921

Abstract

This chapter describes recent research studies about kohlrabi, a versatile vegetable with important health benefits (e.g. reduces risk of breast and prostate cancer, improves body metabolism, helps in weight loss diets, etc.). The investigations are focused on pale-green kohlrabi giving an accurate and precise description, from a qualitative point of view, of the bioactive compounds found in different parts of the pale-green kohlrabi: core, peel, leaves and equal combinations between these parts. All the active principles from pale-green kohlrabi are extracted following a well-established method, in an aqueous medium at a constant temperature of 4°C for 24 h. The qualitative screening of phytochemicals gives details regarding the presence or absence of chemical compounds using different colour reactions.

Keywords: *Brassica oleracea*, kohlrabi, aqueous extracts, bioactive compounds, qualitative screening

1. Introduction

Brassica vegetables, also known as 'cruciferous vegetables', consist of a large group of herbaceous plants that include some of the world's most cultivated vegetables, namely cabbage, broccoli and cauliflower. Besides their main use as food ingredients, *Brassica* vegetables are full of antioxidants that help lower the potential risk of different types of cancers and coronary heart issues and are an important source of vitamin C, folic acid and numerous minerals such as iron, potassium and selenium [1].

Brassicas are also renowned for containing disease-fighting compounds, phytochemicals that occur naturally in plants and exhibit a variety of health benefits for the human body. One of those biologically active compounds is glucosinolates, sulphur-containing phytochemicals with strong anti-cancer properties [2–4]. *Brassica* vegetables contain significant amounts of carotenoids such as zeaxanthin and lutein, two important components of the macula lutea region of the retina, and, therefore, play an important role in the prevention of age-related macular degeneration [5].

Kohlrabi (*Brassica oleracea* of the Gongylodes group) is one of the top vitamin C plants (one cup of kohlrabi contains more than 100% of the daily dose recommended for human consumption). It has European origins, being often called 'German turnip', with a sweet and delicate taste, rather a combination between radish and cabbage.

Kohlrabi is a bulbous vegetable available all year round and can be eaten either raw or cooked; both root and leaves are recommended in human consumption as they contain significant amounts of nutrients and are poor in calories [6, 7].

Several varieties of kohlrabi are commonly grown and commercially available, including White Vienna, Purple Vienna, Grand Duke, Gigante, Purple Danube and White Danube.

The main benefits in human health of kohlrabi are presented in **Figure 1**.

In the present chapter, different parts (e.g. core, peel and leaves) of pale-green kohlrabi are used to prepare five distinct aqueous extracts that are analysed by means of qualitative phytochemical content [8–10].

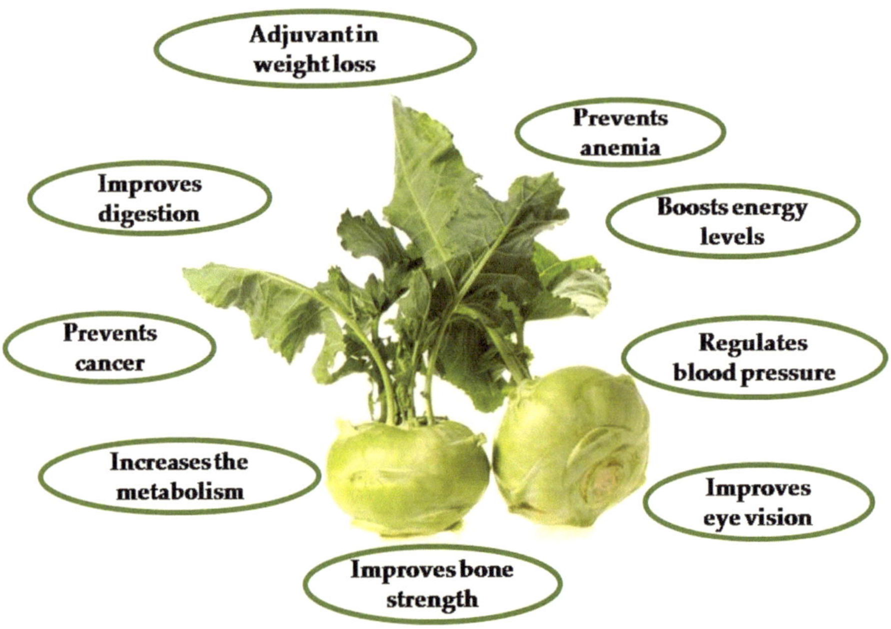

Figure 1. Health benefits of pale green kohlrabi.

http://dx.doi.org/10.5772/intechopen.76921

2. Preparation of aqueous extracts from pale-green kohlrabi

Five distinct aqueous extracts are prepared from different parts of pale-green kohlrabi, as follows:

- three simple aqueous extracts from only one part, for example, core, peel and leaves; and
- two combined aqueous extracts from core and peel in equal parts, respectively core, peel and leaves in equal amounts.

The main steps involved in the preparation of aqueous extracts from pale-green kohlrabi are (**Figure 2**) acquiring pale-green kohlrabi from the local market, thoroughly washing it with tap water once and distilled water thrice, separating the component parts (core, peel, leaves), shade-drying it at room temperature, grinding the components into fine parts, extracting a determined quantity of the dried powder in an aqueous medium for 24 h and filtering the resulting extract until no debris are present in the aqueous extract.

All five distinct pale-green kohlrabi aqueous extracts are prepared according to the same method that was generally described above; the only difference is the amount of dried plant that resulted after the extraction and the volume of the resulting aqueous extract. In **Table 1** the amount of dried plant material before and after the extraction is presented, and **Table 2** contains the exact volume of different resulting aqueous extracts compared to the initial volume of distilled water.

The extractive value (yield percentage) of the kohlrabi (peel, core, leaves, equal amounts of peel and core, equal amounts of peel, core and leaves) samples was calculated before and after

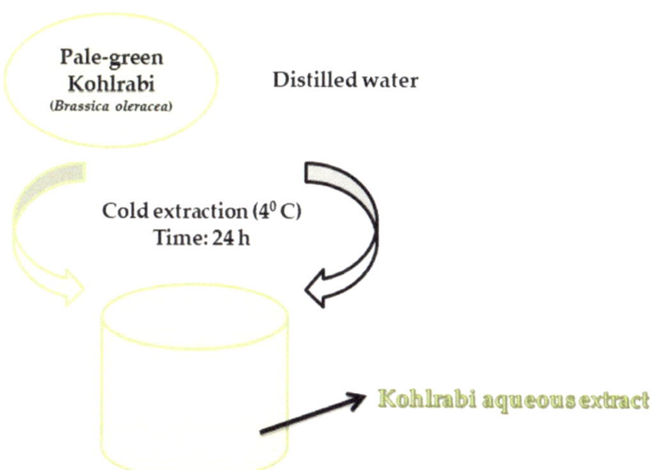

Figure 2. General method for preparation of aqueous extract from pale-green kohlrabi.

Crt. No.	Aqueous extract	Weight before extraction (g)	Weight after extraction (g)	Yield (%)
1	Pale-green kohlrabi core	25	19.06	76.24
2	Pale-green kohlrabi peel	25	21.26	85.04
3	Pale-green kohlrabi leaves	25	20.64	82.56
4	Pale-green kohlrabi core and peel (equal amounts)	25 (12.5 g core + 12.5 g peel)	17.63	70.52
5	Pale-green kohlrabi core, peel and leaves (equal amounts)	30 (10 g core + 10 g peel + 10 g leaves)	22.85	76.17

Table 1. Quantities of solid vegetal material before and after the extraction.

Crt. No.	Aqueous extract	Distilled water (mL)	Volume of aqueous extract (mL)
1	Pale-green kohlrabi core	250	202
2	Pale-green kohlrabi peel	250	170
3	Pale-green kohlrabi leaves	250	192
4	Pale-green kohlrabi core and peel	250	190
5	Pale-green kohlrabi core, peel and leaves	300	208

Table 2. Volume of resulted aqueous extracts from pale green kohlrabi.

the preparation of the aqueous extracts using the formula and the results are also presented in **Table 1** [11]:

$$\text{Extract yield } \% = [W_1/W_2] \times 100.$$

where W_1 = net powder weight (grams) after extraction and W_2 = total powder weight (grams) used for the preparation of aqueous extracts.

3. Qualitative screening of phytochemicals from pale-green kohlrabi aqueous extracts

Various standard qualitative phytochemical analyses are known that allow the determination of chemical groups or compounds in aqueous extracts from different plants. The majority of these qualitative tests is based on the change of colour or precipitation as a clear response to the presence of that specific chemical compound [12, 13]. It is important to mention that these colour reactions allow only to highlight the presence or absence of various chemical groups and not the amount in which they are present in different aqueous extracts.

Standard phytochemical methods are used to analyse from a qualitative point of view all the five aqueous extracts prepared as mentioned in the previous section [14, 15].

3.1. Qualitative screening of carbohydrates

Carbohydrates, the sugars and fibres that can be found in every fruit or vegetable, represent one the basic food groups of great importance for human health. Carbohydrates are among the top three macronutrients, along with protein and fats.

A large number of analytical techniques have been used to determine the concentration and different types of carbohydrates found in foods.

There are four different standard phytochemical methods used for the qualitative screening of carbohydrates found in aqueous extracts [16] (**Table 3**):

a. A 1 ml Molisch reagent (a solution of α-naphthol in ethylic alcohol) is added to 2 ml aqueous extract to which few drops of concentrated sulphuric acid are slowly dripped until a purple-reddish colour appears;

b. To 1 ml of aqueous extract, 5 ml of Benedict's reagent (a complex solution of sodium carbonate, sodium citrate and copper sulphate pentahydrate) was added and boiled for 5 min. The bluish-green colour indicates the presence of carbohydrates;

c. To 1 ml of aqueous extract, few drops of Fehling A reagent (aqueous solution of copper sulphate) are added, which gives green colouration;

d. To 1 ml of aqueous extract, few drops of Fehling B reagent (a solution of potassium sodium tartrate in sodium hydroxide) are added, and a brown colour appears.

It is clear from the colour reaction described above that, with the only exception of pale-green kohlrabi peel, carbohydrates can be found in all the other four aqueous extracts.

3.2. Qualitative screening of tannins and phlobatannins

Tannins are a group of phenol compounds usually found in plants, part of a group of chemicals called 'polyphenols', and almost all of them are soluble in water. Phlobatannins are largely considered a novel class of ring-isomerized condensed tannins [17].

Phytochemical test	Pale-green kohlrabi core	Pale-green kohlrabi peel	Pale-green kohlrabi leaves	Pale-green kohlrabi core and peel	Pale-green kohlrabi core, peel and leaves
Carbohydrates—Molisch	Purple solution	Yellow-mustard solution	Purple solution	Purple solution	Purple solution
Carbohydrates—Benedict	Blue-green solution	Turquoise solution	Blue-green solution	Blue-green solution	Blue-green solution
Carbohydrates—Fehling A	Green solution	Turquoise opalescent solution	Green solution	Green solution	Green solution
Carbohydrates—Fehling B	Brown solution	Citron-yellow solution	Brown solution	Brown solution	Brown solution

Table 3. Qualitative screening of carbohydrates.

Phytochemical test	Pale-green kohlrabi core	Pale-green kohlrabi peel	Pale-green kohlrabi leaves	Pale-green kohlrabi core and peel	Pale-green kohlrabi core, peel and leaves
Tannins	Brown-yellow opalescent solution	Yellow-brown solution	Brown-yellow solution	Brown solution	Brown solution
Phlobatannins	Red-brown opalescent solution	White opalescent solution	Red-brown opalescent solution	Red-brown solution	Yellow solution

Table 4. Qualitative screening of tannins and phlobatannins.

According to the literature [18], the test for tannins consists of the following steps: to 1 ml of aqueous extract 2 ml of 5% ferric chloride is added and a dark blue or greenish black colour appears.

Phlobatannins are tested as follows: To 1 ml of aqueous extract few drops of diluted HCl (1%) are added and a red precipitate appears (**Table 4**).

Tannins are absent from all the five pale-green kohlrabi aqueous extracts while small traces of phlobatannins can be found in three aqueous extracts: pale-green kohlrabi core, pale green kohlrabi leaves and in the aqueous extract prepared from equal amounts of core and peel.

3.3. Qualitative screening of saponins

The general method is 2 ml of aqueous extract and 2 ml of distilled water are shaken in a graduated cylinder for 15 min. A 1 cm foam layer indicates the presence of saponins (see **Table 5**).

3.4. Qualitative screening of flavonoids and phenolic flavonoids

Flavonoids are a class of polyphenolic compounds with important functions in plants: attract pollinating insects, fight against different microbial infections and control cell growth [19].

Flavonoids are tested as follows: 2 ml of aqueous extract and 1 ml of 2 N sodium hydroxide are mixed. A yellow colour indicates the presence of flavonoids. The test for phenolic flavonoids involves the reaction between 1 ml of aqueous extract and 2 ml of 10% lead acetate solution reacting to give a brown precipitate (see **Table 6**).

Flavonoids are present in two aqueous extracts (pale-green kohlrabi peel and pale-green kohlrabi leaves), while phenolic flavonoids occur in pale-green kohlrabi core and in the two complex aqueous extracts that contain it.

Phytochemical test	Pale-green kohlrabi core	Pale-green kohlrabi peel	Pale-green kohlrabi leaves	Pale-green kohlrabi core and peel	Pale-green kohlrabi core, peel and leaves
Saponins	2 cm foam layer	3 cm foam layer	2.5 cm foam layer	3.5 cm foam layer	3 cm foam layer

Table 5. Qualitative screening of saponins.

Phytochemical test	Pale-green kohlrabi core	Pale-green kohlrabi peel	Pale-green kohlrabi leaves	Pale-green kohlrabi core and peel	Pale-green kohlrabi core, peel and leaves
Flavonoids	Red-brown solution	Pale-yellow solution	Pale-yellow opalescent solution	Red-brown solution	Brown solution
Phenolic flavonoids	Brown precipitate	White precipitate	Pale-yellow precipitate	Pale-brown solution	Opalescent brown-yellow solution

Table 6. Qualitative screening of flavonoids and phenolic flavonoids.

3.5. Qualitative screening of alkaloids

Alkaloids are naturally occurring compounds that contain basic nitrogen atoms. They have a large variety of pharmacological applications: antimalaria, antiasthma, anticancer, analgesic, and so on [20].

There are two different standard phytochemical methods:

a. To 1 ml of aqueous extract, 1 ml of Wagner's reagent (iodine in potassium iodide solution) is added leading to the formation of a reddish brown precipitate.

b. To 1 ml of aqueous extract, 2 ml of concentrated hydrochloric acid and a few drops of Mayer reagent are added, resulting in a green colour or white precipitate (the results are presented in **Table 7**).

According to the results presented in **Table 7**, alkaloids are absent from all the aqueous extracts from pale-green kohlrabi, whatever method was used for the qualitative screening.

3.6. Qualitative screening of anthraquinones and anthocyanosides

The standard method used for the qualitative screening of anthraquinones involves the reaction of 1 ml of aqueous extract with a few drops of 10% ammonia solution, leading to the formation of a pink precipitate. Anthocyanosides are observed when 1 ml of aqueous extract is mixed with 5 ml of dilute hydrochloric acid and a pink colour appears (see **Table 8** for the results).

Phytochemical test	Pale-green kohlrabi core	Pale-green kohlrabi peel	Pale-green kohlrabi leaves	Pale-green kohlrabi core and peel	Pale-green kohlrabi core, peel and leaves
Alkaloids—Wagner	Opalescent red-brown solution	Opalescent brown solution	Opalescent yellow-brown solution	Clear red-brown solution	Opalescent red-brown solution
Alkaloids—Mayer	Opalescent orange-yellow solution	Opalescent beige solution	Brown-yellow opalescent solution	Red-brown solution	Opalescent beige solution

Table 7. Qualitative screening of alkaloids.

Phytochemical test	Pale-green kohlrabi core	Pale-green kohlrabi peel	Pale-green kohlrabi leaves	Pale-green kohlrabi core and peel	Pale-green kohlrabi core, peel and leaves
Anthraquinones	Red-beige solution	Pale-yellow opalescent solution	Green-yellow precipitate	Opalescent red-brown solution	Opalescent red-beige solution
Anthocyanosides	Red-yellow opalescent solution	Yellow opalescent solution	Pale-pink opalescent solution	Orange-red solution	Pale-beige solution

Table 8. Qualitative screening of anthraquinones and anthocyanosides.

Phytochemical test	Pale-green kohlrabi core	Pale-green kohlrabi peel	Pale-green kohlrabi leaves	Pale-green kohlrabi core and peel	Pale-green kohlrabi core, peel and leaves
Proteins and aminoacids—Millon	Red-beige solution	Opalescent White solution, pale-yellow after heating	Opalescent beige solution, brown after heating	White brown solution, beige-red after heating	Opalescent beige solution, red-brown after heating
Proteins and aminoacids—Biuret test	Red-yellow opalescent solution	Opalescent blue solution	Green-yellow solution, blue precipitate	Dark-brown solution	Violet-green solution

Table 9. Qualitative screening of proteins and aminoacids.

3.7. Qualitative screening of proteins and aminoacids

There are two different standard methods used (see results in **Table 9**):

a. 1 ml of aqueous extract reacts with 5–6 drops of Millon's reagent, and a white precipitate appears that changes its colour to red upon heating;

b. To 3 ml of aqueous extract, 3 ml of 4% sodium hydroxide solution and few drops of 1% copper sulphate are added to form a purple solution.

3.8. Qualitative screening of steroids and terpenoids

The general procedure to test the presence of steroids is To 1 ml of aqueous extract, add 10 ml of chloroform and slowly drip 10 ml of sulphuric acid. The upper layer turns red and the sulphuric acid layer turns yellow green. Similarly, terpenoids are analysed by reacting 1 ml of aqueous extract with 2 ml of chloroform and then slowly few drops of concentrated sulphuric acid. An interface with a reddish brown colouration appears (**Table 10**).

The qualitative screening of steroids revealed that these phytochemicals are absent from all the extracts while very small traces of terpenoids could be visually observed in three aqueous extracts: pale-green kohlrabi core and the other two extracts that contain this part.

Phytochemical test	Pale-green kohlrabi core	Pale-green kohlrabi peel	Pale-green kohlrabi leaves	Pale-green kohlrabi core and peel	Pale-green kohlrabi core, peel and leaves
Steroids	Colourless layer, brown ring, colourless layer	Colourless layer, beige ring, colourless layer	Colourless layer, light-brown ring, colourless layer, brown ring	Colourless layer, brown ring, colourless layer	Colourless layer, brown ring, colourless layer
Terpenoids	Colourless layer, yellow-brown ring	Colourless layer, white ring (precipitate)	Pale-yellow layer, beige ring	Yellow-brown layer, red-brown ring	Colourless layer, brown-yellow opalescent ring

Table 10. Qualitative screening of steroids and terpenoids.

3.9. Qualitative screening of cardiac glycosides

There are two different standard phytochemical methods:

a. 1 ml of aqueous extract, 1 ml of $FeCl_3$ reagent (1 ml of 5% $FeCl_3$ solution mixed with 99 ml of glacial acetic acid) and few drops of concentrated H_2SO_4 gives a greenish-blue colour that appears in time;

b. 5 ml of aqueous extract, 2 ml of glacial acetic acid, a drop of $FeCl_3$ solution and 1 ml of concentrated H_2SO_4 forms a brown ring and often a purple ring appears below (see results in **Table 11**).

Regardless of the method used in the screening, cardiac glycosides are absent from all the aqueous extracts prepared from pale-green kohlrabi.

Phytochemical test	Pale-green kohlrabi core	Pale-green kohlrabi peel	Pale-green kohlrabi leaves	Pale-green kohlrabi core and peel	Pale-green kohlrabi core, peel and leaves
Cardiac glycosides—$FeCl_3$ reagent	Colourless layer, thin brown ring, beige clear solution	Colourless clear layer, yellow suspension	Colourless layer, pink-beige suspension	Colourless layer, brown ring, opalescent beige layer	Colourless layer, opalescent yellow-beige ring
Cardiac glycosides—Keller-Killani test	Colourless layer, brown ring, beige opalescent layer, red opalescent layer	Colourless layer, red-beige opalescent solution	Colourless layer, yellow-brown layer, brown-red layer	Colourless layer, brown ring, red-brown layer, beige precipitate layer	Colourless layer, brown ring, red-brown layer

Table 11. Qualitative screening of cardiac glycosides.

4. Conclusions

This chapter describes the qualitative phytochemical screening of five distinct aqueous extracts prepared from different parts of pale-green kohlrabi, a versatile vegetable part of *Brassica* genus with numerous benefits for human health. The qualitative screening is achieved by standard methods that are able to determine whether a phytochemical is present or not in a specific aqueous extract.

The qualitative screening of carbohydrates revealed that, except for pale-green kohlrabi peel aqueous extract, in all the other extracts carbohydrates are present. It can be clearly stated that tannins are absent from all the five pale-green kohlrabi aqueous extracts. Phlobatannins can be found, in small traces, in three aqueous extracts: pale-green kohlrabi core, pale-green kohlrabi leaves and in the aqueous extract prepared from equal amounts of core and peel.

In smaller or larger quantities, saponins are present in all five aqueous extracts, according to the height of the resulting foam layer, while alkaloids, cardiac glycosides and steroids are clearly absent from all the extracts.

Acknowledgements

This paper received the financial support of the projects: PN 120BG/2016 and PN 18.22.04.01.01.

Conflict of interest

The authors declare no potential conflicts of interest with respect to the research, authorship and publication of this article.

Author details

Ana-Alexandra Sorescu[1,2]*, Alexandrina Nuta[1,3] and Rodica-Mariana Ion[1,2]

*Address all correspondence to: anaalexandrasorescu@yahoo.com

1 The National Research and Development Institute for Chemistry and Petrochemistry—ICECHIM, Evaluation and Conservation of Cultural Heritage, Bucharest, Romania

2 Valahia University, Materials Engineering Doctoral School, Targoviste, Romania

3 The Romanian Academy, "Stefan S. Nicolau" Institute of Virology, Bucharest, Romania

References

[1] Martinez-Espla A, Zapata PJ, Castillo S, Guillen F, Martinez-Romero F, Valero D, Serrano M. Preharvest application of methyl jasmonate (MeJA) in two plum cultivars. 1. Improvement of fruit growth and quality attributes at harvest. Postharvest Biology and Technology. 2014;**98**:98-105

[2] Macleod G, Macleod AJ. The glucosinolates and aroma volatiles of green kohlrabi. Phytochemistry. 1990;**29**:1183-1187. DOI: 10.1016/0031-9422(90)85425-F

[3] Wiebe HJ, Habegger R, Liebig HP. Quantification of vernalization and devernalization effects for kohlrabi (*Brassica oleracea* convar. Acephala var. gongylodes L.). Scientia Horticulturae. 1992;**50**:11-20. DOI: 10.1016/S0304-4238(05)80004-4

[4] Escalona VH, Aguayo E, Artes F. Metabolic activity and quality changes of whole and fresh-cut kohlrabi (*Brassica oleracea* L. *gongylodes* group) stored under controlled atmosphere. Postharvest Biology and Technology. 2006;**41**:181-190. DOI: 10.1016/j.postharvbio.2006.04.001

[5] Thomas RA, Krishnakumari S. Phytochemical profiling of *Myristica fragrans* seed extract with different organic solvents. Journal of Pharmaceutical and Clinical Research. 2015;**1**:304-307

[6] Caroling G, Vinodhini E, Mercy Ranjitham A, Shanti P. Biosynthesis of copper nanoparticles using *Phyllanthus embilica* (gooseberry) extract—Characterisation and study of antimicrobial effects. International Jorunal of Nanomaterials and Chemistry. 2015;**1**:53-63

[7] Veerachari U, Bopaiah AK. Preliminary phyto-chemical evaluation of the leaf extract of five *Cassia* Species. Journal of Chemical and Pharmaceutical Research. 2011;**5**:574-583

[8] Periannan U, Pragakaran G. Studies on antibacterial activity and preliminary phytochemical analysisof *Aegle marmelos* L. (Beal). International Journal of Current Sciences and Technology. 2013;**2**:17-20

[9] Subhash CM, Vivekananda M. Essentials of Botanical Extractions. Principles and Applications. 1st ed. San Diego, United States: Elsevier Science Publishing Co Inc. 2015;173-185. DOI: 10.1016/B978-0-12-802325-9.00009-4

[10] Escalona VH, Aguayo E, Artes F. Modified atmosphere packaging improved quality of kohlrabi stems. LWT-Food Science and Technology. 2007;**40**(3):397-403. DOI: 10.1016/j.lwt.2006.02.006

[11] Gong R, Zhang X, Liu H, Sun Y, Liu B. Uptake of cationic dyes from aqueous solution by biosorption onto granular kohlrabi peel. Bioresource Technology. 2007;**98**(6):1319-1323. DOI: 10.1016/j.biortech.2006.04.034

[12] Fahey JW. Reference Module in Food Science. Encyclopedia of Food and Health. 1st ed. Kidlington, Oxford: Elsevier Ltd; 2016. 469 p. DOI: 10.1016/B978-0-12-384947-2.00083-0

[13] Choi S, Beuchat LR, Kim H, Ryu JH. Viability of sprout seeds as affected by treatment with aqueous chlorine dioxide and dry heat, and reduction of *Escherichia coli* O157:H7 and *Salmonella enterica* on pak choi seeds by sequential treatment with chlorine dioxide, drying and dry heat. Food Microbiology. 2016;**54**:127-132. DOI: 10.1016/j.fm.2015.10.007

[14] Kosewski G, Gorna I, Boleslawska I, Kowalowka M, Wieckowska B, Glowska AK, Morawska A, Jakubowski K, Dobrzynska M, Miszczuk P, Przyslawski J. Comparison of antioxidative properties of raw vegetables and thermally processed ones using the conventional and sous-vide methods. Food Chemistry. 2018;**240**:1092-1096. DOI: 10.1016/j.foodchem.2017.08.048

[15] Muhamad II, Hassan ND, Mamat SNH, Nawi NM, Rashid WA, Tan NA. Extraction technologies and solvents of phytocompounds from plant materials: Physicochemical characterization and identification of ingredients and bioactive compounds from plant extracts using various instrumentation. Ingredients Extraction by Physicochemical Methods in Food. Handbook of Food Bioengineering. 1st ed. London: Elsevier Ltd. 2017. 523 p. DOI: 10.1016/B978-0-12-811521-3.00014-4

[16] Picariello L, Gambuti A, Picariello B, Moio L. Evolution of pigments, tannins and acetaldehyde during forced oxidation of red wine: Effects of tannins addition. LWT. 2017;**77**:370-375. DOI: 10.1016/j.lwt.2016.11.064

[17] Steenkamp JA, Steynberg JP, Brandt EV, Roux DV. Phlobatannins, a novel class of ring-isomerized condensed tannins. Journal of the Chemical Society, Chemical Communications. 1985. DOI: 10.1039/c39850001678

[18] Loman AA, Ju LK. Enzyme-based processing of soybean carbohydrate: Recent developments and future prospects. Enzyme and Microbial Technology. 2017;**106**:35-47. DOI: 10.1016/j.enzmictec.2017.06.013

[19] Flavonoids [Internet]. Available from: http://lpi.oregonstate.edu/mic/dietary-factors/phytochemicals/flavonoids [Accessed: March 25, 2018]

[20] Tadeusz A. Alkaloids-Secrets of Life. Amsterdam: Elsevier; 2007

Chapter 5

Agronomic Factors Influencing *Brassica* Productivity and Phytochemical Quality

Cristine Vanz Borges, Santino Seabra Junior,
Franciely S. Ponce and Giuseppina Pace Pereira Lima

Additional information is available at the end of the chapter

http://dx.doi.org/10.5772/intechopen.74732

Abstract

Agronomic practices and climatic factors affect the content and profile of phytochemicals. The effects of the environment, such as salinity, climate, and other abiotic factors, promote biochemical responses, inducing changes in the quantity and quality of polyphenol compounds, carotenoids, vitamins, glucosinolates, and polyamines, which are bioactive compounds. In plants, among the various functions, some phytochemicals can protect against biotic factors. *Brassica* vegetables are a source of several primary and secondary metabolism compounds, and they might be responsible for disease prevention. In addition, the increase of bioactive compounds in plant-based foods is important to the diet and consequently for the improvement of public health. In this chapter, we will point out the abiotic factors that affect the productive performance, quality, and chemical composition of different *Brassica* species and cultivars. We will also discuss its implications on plant protection and human health.

Keywords: environmental factors, cultivation conditions, polyphenol, carotenoids, glucosinolates

1. Introduction

The *Brassica* ceae family, previously known as Cruciferae, is composed of 338 genus and around 3700 species. The family includes many plants of economic importance, for the production of edible oil, such as the canola, forage rape (*Brassica napus*), and seasoning plants, as the mustard and also various species for consumption, in which the leaf, stem, roots, and tubercles are edible parts. The main genus, *Brassica*, is formed by 37 species, which can be annual and biannual, including even weeds, wild plants, and domestic crops. *Brassica* vegetables originate from regions between the Mediterranean and the Sahara, where the climate consists of mild winters followed by hot and dry summers. Besides that, there are species inside the genus that are well adapted to colder regions, and many species are now considered naturalized in the entire world and are commonly observed in Western Europe, in the Mediterranean, and in temperate regions of Asia. In addition, many species also grow in as invasive weeds in the Americas (North and South) and Australasia [1].

The species of the *Brassica* genus were widely modified and domesticated by human beings and are vegetables cultivated worldwide [2], especially the varieties belonging to the species *Brassica oleracea*, which includes cabbage, tronchuda cabbage (*Brassica oleracea* L. var. costata DC), mustard, rocket, and Brussels sprout (*Brassica oleracea* L. var. gemmifera), among others (**Figure 1**). Among these species, we also found broccoli, where the most consumed part is the inflorescence, the cauliflower, from which the floral peduncle is consumed and the tubercles, as the radish and the turnip.

Brassica vegetables have attracted great attention due to the presence of phytochemicals with recognized beneficial functions in the human organism, reducing the risk of diseases [3]. These vegetables are potential sources of anticarcinogenic and antioxidant compounds as the glucosinolates (GLS), vitamin C, phenolic acids, flavonols, anthocyanidins, carotenoids, and amino acids [4]. Most of the researches are focused on the content of secondary metabolites, mainly the glucosinolates. The benefits to human health from the ingestion of these vegetables, such as the reduced risk of degenerative diseases, are in great part attributed to the content of secondary metabolites substances of the plants [5]. Besides the human health aspects, these metabolites play a fundamental role in the plants' defense against microorganisms, raising the interest in higher quantities of these secondary compounds as a strategy of increasing the protection of the cultures and reducing the use of agrochemicals.

Variations in the agronomic conditions (e.g., vegetal species, cultivars, development stage, plants organs, fertilization, and soil pH) and climatic factors (e.g., light intensity and water availability) are known for significantly affecting the phytochemical content and profile. The understanding of the effects of climatic and agronomic factors is necessary for increasing the predictability of the desired compounds, increasing the benefits related to the human health and to the plants' protection (plague control) [6]. Although there is little information on the real influence of cultivation on the contents of glucosinolates and other important phytochemicals in *Brassicas*, it appears that the use of ecological practices can induce a rise in the content of these molecules. In this chapter, we provide a general view about the roles of the glucosinolates and other phytochemicals present in *Brassicaceae* and their implications in the plants' protection, productivity, and human health, as well as emphasize the factors that affect the contents of these compounds in *Brassica* vegetables.

http://dx.doi.org/10.5772/intechopen.74732

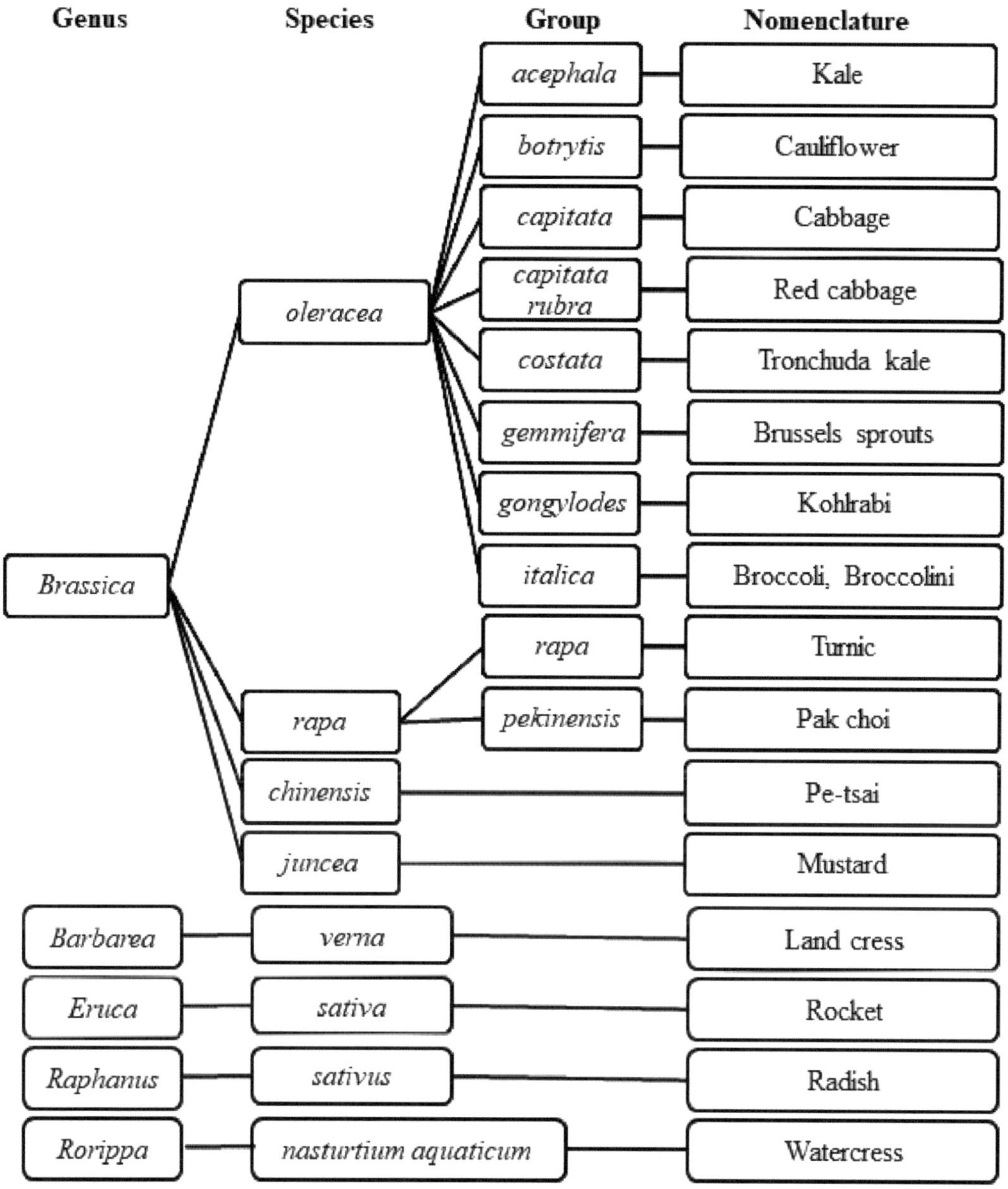

Figure 1. Main *brassicas* cultivated worldwide.

2. Agronomic factors and production

The photosynthetic activity is the base for the production of reserves in the plant, which will constitute the biomass, a factor that can determine the vegetal development limits. The production depends on the interaction between the productive potential and the environmental factors. The edaphoclimatic factors are directly related to productive responses that influence the flowering, hydric balance, respiration, and absorption of minerals. Latitude, altitude, rainfall, topography, and soil physics act indirectly on the production and other factors, such as solar radiation, temperature, water, and chemical elements of the soil act directly on the photosynthesis. The environmental factors, such as water, temperature, quality, and quantity of light hours, will determine the plants' growth rate.

The temperature is a climatic factor that can limit the production of determined species in tropical and equatorial regions. Besides determining the growth and development, it establishes the end of the vegetative stage and the beginning of the productive stage in the biennial species, such as broccoli, cauliflower, Brussels sprout, among other species. The broccoli has a better productive development under average temperatures between 60 and 65°F, with a maximum of 75°F [7]. Prolonged periods of temperature above 77°C can retard the formation of inflorescence in plants that are in phase of vegetative growth, reducing the size and causing the development of leaves and bracts in the floral peduncles [8].

The temperature strongly influences the plants' metabolic activity, and the stress caused by high and low temperatures can induce effects in the primary and secondary metabolism (**Table 1**). The heat or cold can affect the membrane fluidity, metabolism, and cytoskeleton rearrangement, consequently affecting the vegetative and reproductive tissues [9]. Abrupt increases of temperature can provoke excessively fast growth of the inflorescence and elongating the peduncle in certain cultivars [10]. Cultivations in conditions of high temperatures, where there are only few days with ideal temperatures for vernalization, the plants can continue to vegetate or to not produce commercial inflorescences, which means uneven bunches, the presence of bracts, and low compactness of the head and yellow coloration. Temperatures below the ideal level can prolong the cycle of provoke premature flowering in some species, as in the case of summer cauliflowers submitted to low temperatures [11]. Among the *brassicas* more tolerant to the cold, the minimum temperature for the germination and cultivation for species is 40°F and the maximum tolerated temperature can reach 105°F for turnip and kohlrabi, which are the most tolerant species to temperature in the germination phase. However, in the cultivation phase, the maximum temperature is situated around 75°F. In Brazil, some regions with mild temperatures and with mensal averages varying from 66 to 88°F, there are reports of commercial cultivation of broccoli, kale, rocket, and watercress [12]. However, cauliflower, cabbage, and radish are also cultivated in tropical regions. These cultivations are favored by the utilization of thermotolerant cultivars obtained by genetic improvement.

The plants can be modified to some degree, tolerating light stresses from either low or high temperatures when slowly submitted to the stress, leading to acclimatization. By contrast, plants that survive the exposition to conditions above the ideal temperature can produce chaperones, molecules that are related to the antioxidant activity, and solutes accumulation [9]. Low temperatures cause reduction in the enzymatic activity, rigidity of membranes, destabilization of protein complexes, compromise of photosynthesis, and rupture of the membranes. Cellular alterations associated to the tolerance to cold and/or freezing include the accumulation of sugar or compatible solutes, changes in the membrane composition, and synthesis of dehydrin-like proteins [9].

The stress by temperature can cause changes in the plants' chemical constitution. Broccoli sprouts present increased glucosinolate contents when cultivated under high (84.2 or 89.6°F) or low temperatures (51.8 or 60.8°F), comparing the cultivated sprouts under ideal temperature (70.7°F) [13]. Similar to the sprouts, the broccoli leaves showed the highest glucosinolate level when cultivated under 53.6 or 89.6°F. This effect was also observed in younger cabbage plants. Under low temperatures, there is an increase of the glucosinolate levels in broccoli and watercress (**Table 1**). The combination of temperature and precipitation influences the

Stress factor		Productive and/or biochemical response	Citations
Temperature	Heat	Affects the glucosinolates content	[59]
		Higher glucosinolates production	[13]
	Cold	Higher glucosinolates production	[13]
		Higher glucosinolates production in broccoli under low temperatures	[60]
	Thermal amplitude	Higher glucosinolates production in broccoli plants under temperatures between 53.6 and 89.6°F, compared to plants under temperature 71.6F	[61]
Luminosity	Competition (population density and consortium)	Reduced levels of trypsin inhibitors in *Brassica napus* seedlings	[6]
		Reduced levels of glucosinolates in the leaves and roots in *B. napus*	
	Excess	Photoinhibition, thermal stress, and stomatal closing, leading to a reduction of net photosynthesis in *brassicas*, included *B. napus*.	[62]
	Protected cultivation (light diffusion and shading)	Mustard plants (*B. juncea*) cultivated under shading screens of 50% showed lower quantities of ascorbic acid, larger foliar area, chlorophyll, carotenoids, N, NO_3, and a higher content of mineral nutrients in comparison to the complete solar luminosity	[63]
	Photoperiod	Affects the glucosinolates content	[59]
		Spring broccoli growth in intermediate temperatures, high luminous intensity, longer days, and dry conditions have the highest total GLS content	[6] [61]
		Glucosinolates levels in kale are not influenced by the photoperiod	
Water	Hydric restriction	Growth reduction, lower yield of cabbage heads, and an increase of dry mass	[64]
		Kale: growth reduction, biomass reduction, increase of sorbitol, sucrose, verbascose and kestose levels, and a decrease of manitol	[65] [66] [67]
		An increase in the sugar content in the phloem sap of broccoli submitted at hydric stress	
		Lower glucosinolate content in broccoli in hydric restriction	
		Biomass reduction, an increase of nitrogen in the leaf, and a darker green leaf in Chinese cabbage	

Stress factor		Productive and/or biochemical response	Citations
Salinity		Growth reduction, Na or Cl accumulation, and lower productivity	[68]
		A decrease of fresh matter in the aerial part of broccoli	[69]
		An increase in GLS content and phenolic compounds	[70]
		A drastic decrease in the vitamin C content in old broccoli leaves	[71]
		A significant decrease in the vitamin C content in young broccoli leaves;	[72]
		Loss of flavonoids in old broccoli leaves;	
		Loss of turgor	
		Accumulation of glucosinolates in *B. napus* L.;	
		Reduction in the nitrate content	
		Increase or no effect in the nitrate content	
Fertilization	Nitrogen (N)	Nitrogen fertilization influences the GLS metabolism in broccoli	[73]
	Sulfur (S)	High level of sulfur provided an increase of polyphenol contents (flavonoids and phenolic acids) in *B. rapa* ssp. *sylvestris*	[74]
		An increase of the total glucosinolates with the increase of fertilization with sulfur	[75]
		Higher quantities of sulfur and nitrogen combined did not provide higher contents of glucosinolates	[60]

Table 1. Effect of environmental factors in the production and biochemical compounds in *brassicas*.

glucosinolate content in *brassicas* (white cabbage, red cabbage, savoy cabbage, Brussels sprouts, cauliflower, kale, kohlrabi, turnip, red radish, black radish, and white radish). High and low precipitations induce higher contents of glucosinolates, when compared to the same vegetables cultivated in a year with mild temperatures and higher precipitation [14].

The light is a factor that influences the *brassicas*' performance. The increase in the luminous intensity corresponds to a rise in the photosynthetic activity (within certain limits), while the decrease promotes a higher cellular elongation, resulting in etiolated plants. However, this response depends on the species' susceptibility and on the plants' density, producing a competition for light or on excessive shading obtained by the use of screens. The amount of energy intercepted is dependent on the characteristics of the cultivation system, row spacing, consortium, and even the architecture characteristics of each genotype, such as the leaf inclination. In the same plant it is possible to occur leaves exposed or not to the sun and with different quantic necessities, with different photosynthetic performance. In this context, there are species that show lower or higher stress when cultivated in a lower spacing or cultivated under consortium. In Ethiopian kale (*B. carinata*) and African nightshade (*Solanum scabrum*), cultivated in consortium and in ideal condition of irrigation and under hydric stress, there was an increase in the glucosinolates content in kale and the maintenance of the biomass production and nutritional characteristics. In addition, low irrigation induced the carotene levels in African nightshade, both under hydric stress and stress provided by the consortium. In opposition, hydric stress did not affect the glucosinolate content in *B. carinata* and the indole glucosinolates in *B. rapa* ssp. Rapifera [15]. These results suggest that the responses to drought and glucosinolates concentration can vary depending on the genotype.

3. *Brassicas'* phytochemical composition

Brassica vegetables are important sources of fibers, vitamins, and minerals. In addition, these vegetables are potential sources of anti-carcinogenic and antioxidant compounds, such as the glucosinolates, vitamin C, phenolic acids, flavonols, anthocyanidins, carotenoids, and amino acids [4]. Most of the current researches are focused on the content of secondary metabolites, mainly of glucosinolates. Many epidemiologic studies indicate that a high ingestion of *brassicaceous* vegetables is associated to a reduced risk of cancer [5, 16], cardiovascular diseases [17], gut diseases (e.g., colite) [18], [19], and diabetes [20].

Many epidemiologic studies do not differ among the types of cruciferous vegetables, but the most common studies in the entire world include the broccoli, cauliflower, cabbages, bok choy, kale, watercress, turnip, and rocket [21]. Besides human health aspects, these metabolites play a fundamental role in the plants' defense against microorganisms; thus, there is an increasing interest in raising the content of these secondary compounds as a strategy of increasing the protection to cultures and reducing the use of agrochemicals.

Even though there is little information on the real influence of the cultivation in the levels of glucosinolates and other important phytochemicals in *brassicas*, it seems that the use of ecological practices can induce a raise of these molecules. In addition, in most cases, it is fundamental to also study the impact of storage and cooking in these compounds, since *brassicas* are not consumed immediately after the harvest, in order to know the real benefits of these vegetables to the human health.

3.1. Glucosinolates

Brassica vegetables are the major source of glucosinolates that has been associated to its bioactivity, and these compounds may be responsible for their observed protecting effects. The glucosinolates are found in 16 families of dicotyledonous plants and in at least 120 different chemical structures that have been identified until now [21]. Depending on the chemical structure of the precursor amino acid, they are now classified into three groups: aliphatic, indole, and aromatic glucosinolates.

The glucosinolates profile and its modifications, together with specific products of hydrolyzation, are being discussed as a plant defense mechanism to deal with various abiotic and biotic stresses. Recent studies showed that glucosinolates, for example, breakdown products of 1-methoxy-indol-3-ylmethyl glucosinolate and 5-phenylpentyl isothiocyanate, exert mutagenic or genotoxic effects in mammalian and bacterial cell studies [22]. Studies indicate that broccoli sprouts are sources of GLS (varying from 679.01 to 554.90 mg/100 g FW), and the predominant GLS is the glucosinolate glucoraphanin (GRA) (33% of the total GLS) [23].

Glucosinolates and isothiocyanates (products of glucosinolate hydrolysis) are produced by some plants in response to biotic stress. They are important as protective agents of the plants, due to their toxic or repelling effects against potential plagues (herbivores, bacteria, and fungi) [24]. Even though these compounds can be used as protection agents in plants, with a great importance in agriculture and horticulture, they are significantly important to human nutrition, due to the preventive effects on human health [24, 25]. These compounds are known for protecting against cancer in humans [26] and, in plants, these secondary metabolites and/or their breakdown products have different biological functions, like fungicidal, bactericidal, nematocidal, and allelopathic properties [27].

Thus, factors influencing phytochemical content and profile in the production of *brassicaceous* plants are worth considering for both plant and human health. There are studies showing that the consumption of *brassica* vegetables has a direct relationship with cancer incidence reduction [28]. Besides GLS, these vegetables contain myrosinase, a thioglucoside glycohydrolase (EC 3.2.3.1) which is released from intracellular compartments when the vegetable tissue is damaged by cutting or chewing and induces GLS hydrolysis into isothiocyanates and nitriles, as the most important products. Sulforaphane is one of the investigated isothiocyanates and is particularly abundant in broccoli var. *italica* in the form of its corresponding glucosinolate glucoraphanin (GRA) (4-methylsulfinylbutyl glucosinolate) [29]. GRA can be converted into sulforaphane and glucobrassicin to indolyl-3-carbinol; both hydrolyzed derivatives are active against carcinogenesis as demonstrated by many *in vitro* experiments or *in vivo* studies [28, 30].

The quality and quantity of GLS differ among the plants species, among the different plant organs (tubercle or leaves), and in function of the ontogeny. The profile of these compounds is not only determined by the plant genetic constitution but also influenced by the environmental conditions [31]. Generally, high levels of GLS occur in response to temperature [32], exposition to different wavelengths [33], nutrients availability [34], and signaling molecules as the salicylic acid (SA) [25], jasmonic acid (JA), and methyl jasmonate (MeJA) [31, 35]. Exogenous applications of SA and its analogous acids, damage by herbivory or treatment with JA, induce increases of indole GLS in *B. napus* [36], *B. campestris* [37], and *B. juncea* [35]. Microorganism infection and/or mechanical damages can promote the biosynthesis of indole GLS and aromatic 2-phenylethyl GLS in *B. rapa* through synthesizing molecules (e.g., methyl jasmonate or jasmonic acid) [31]. In addition, many compounds such as phenolics, terpenoids, and compounds containing sulfur also regulate the biosynthesis [38].

Saline stress (150 mM NaCl) can reduce the total GLS levels, due to the decrease of both aliphatic GLP, as indole (GBS and MBGS), in broccoli sprouts [23]. This decrease is attributed to cell damages induced by Na accumulation [39]. However, studies with broccoli sprouts determined that the decrease in the GLS level in response to excessive contents of NaCl (44% in comparison to the control—0 mM NaCl) can be decreased by the application of MeJA, applied daily from the third day of growth of 10-day-old broccoli sprouts [23].

Brassica foods (e.g., cabbage, cauliflower, broccoli, Brussels sprouts, turnips, and kale) are consumed raw, frozen, or after domestic thermal processing (cooking). Generally, the conventional cooking methods, such as boiling, steaming, pressure cooking, and microwaving, reduce the content of glucosinolates to approximately 30–60%, depending on the method and analyzed compound [40]. Leaves (turning greens) and young-sprouting shoots (turning tops) of *B. rapa* cooked in steam showed maintenance of GLS content, compared to raw vegetable, by preventing leaching and solubilization of these metabolites. By contrast, conventional boiling and high-pressure cooking methods induced losses of GLS levels (64%), and the degradation of different GLS classes (e.g., aliphatic or indolic) was similar in both cooking methods [40]. However, some compounds with important pharmacologic activities can be formed after the thermal processing by hydrolysis (e.g., 2-aminothiophene and dimeric 1,4-dithiane-2,5-di-acetonitrile), increasing the bioactive potential in *brassica* vegetables [41].

The thermal treatment causes denaturation of enzymes that catalyze the degradation of nutrients and some metabolites. When *brassica* vegetables are chopped, ground, or chewed, there is a rupture of the tissues, and the GLSs enter in contact with the myrosinase, inducing the conversion to isothiocyanates, nitriles, thiocyanates, epithionitriles, oxazolidine-2-thiones, and epithioalkanes [42]. The hydrolysis products, mainly during the storage and processing, as well as the myrosinase activity of the gut microbiota, can affect the total content and bioavailability of these compounds [26]. In addition, the glucosinolates are water-soluble compounds and are generally lost by leaching, in methods that use water for cooking.

3.2. Polyphenols

The phenolic compounds are a group of secondary metabolites present in the vegetal kingdom. The most disseminated and diversified groups of polyphenols are the flavonoids, which have C6-C3-C6 flavone skeleton. The flavonoids are important phenolic phytochemicals containing a basic structure of two aromatic benzene rings separated by a heterocyclic-oxygenated ring [43]. The flavonoids and the hydroxycinnamic acids are widely distributed in plants and are important bioactive compounds in the human diet. The dietetic flavonoids have antiviral, anti-inflammatory, antihistaminic, and antioxidant properties. Flavonoids and phenolic acids are the most characterized groups of phenolic compounds in *brassicas* and can protect the plants against UV radiation, microorganisms, and predator insects [44]. In cabbage, many (poly)phenolic compounds were identified, including myricetin, quercetin, kaempferol, luteolin, delphinidin, cyanidin, and pelargonidin [45].

Generally, the phenolic compounds are produced through the phenylpropanoid pathway. Biotic or abiotic stresses, such as elicitors, were reported for inducing alterations in the phenolic compounds contents, as described in broccoli sprouts [23, 46]. In addition, the quality and quantity of the phenols differ among the plant species and among the plant organs. For example, broccoli sprouts have higher phenolic levels (1133.85 mg/100 g FW), when compared with mature broccoli inflorescences (63.4 mg/100 g FW) [45]. Most of the phenolic compounds present in broccoli sprouts are the hydroxycinnamic acids (sinapic acid derivatives), approximately 98% of the total phenolics found [23].

In saline-stress conditions, there is a possibility for a decrease to occur up to 30% in the phenolic compounds' content in *brassicas* (e.g., broccoli sprout). It is important to highlight that the increase or decrease of these compounds in this situation depends on the plant sensibility to salt and on the development stage when the plant was submitted to the stress [23]. The exogenous application of elicitors can also induce the phenolic compounds' biosynthesis, affecting the contents of antioxidant and nutritional compounds in *brassicas*. This technique can be a viable tool to obtain vegetables with higher levels of these bioactive compounds. Studies with broccoli sprouts showed that the prolonged application of low concentrations of SA and MeJA during the sprouting significantly increased the content of phenolic compounds. Exogenous SA (50 μM) applied for 5 days or 100 μM SA for 7 days achieved flavonoids-enriched broccoli sprouts by 24 and 33%, respectively. A 10 μM MeJA was a highly efficient treatment, promoting increases of 31 and 23% in the concentration of flavonoids and total phenolics, respectively [47].

The culinary process is a source of several alterations, both physical and biochemical, modifying the phytochemical constituents present in the vegetables, resulting in changes in the nutritional values [48] of *brassicas*. During the cooking process, the phenolic compounds are highly reactive and can be significantly modified, including the release of conjugated compounds (bound forms), oxidation, degradation, and polymerization [49]. Generally, the effect of boiling in *brassica* vegetables can lead to significant polyphenol losses. During the boiling, because the phenolic compounds are water-soluble, there might be losses by leaching, besides the breaking of these compounds during the thermal processing. The analysis of the water used in experiments with boiled *brassica* vegetables (e.g., in watercress) shows the presence of total phenols in the water (9.35 ± 0.12 mg GAE/g DW), confirming the loss by leaching (raw watercress – 14.86 ± 2.02 mg GAE/g DW). The quantity of phenols found in the water and in cooked material (residual phenols) is not different from the quantity present in raw watercress [50]. In opposition, in these studies, a minimum deleterious effect was demonstrated when microwaving and steaming were used in the content of phenolic compounds. This minimum effect occurs according to the quantity of water used and to the inactivation of oxidative enzymes, which prevent the rupture and the degradation of the phenolic biosynthesis [50].

3.3. Carotenoids

Carotenoids are a class of phytonutrients that are responsible for the colors red, orange, and light yellow in many vegetables and fruits. Most of the *brassica* vegetables contain carotenoids, such as β-carotene, lutein, zeaxanthin, neoxanthin, violaxanthin, and folate, which have important antioxidant, anticarcinogenic properties, and provitamin A [51]. Carotenoids have shown to have functions during the photosynthesis and show an important role in defense mechanisms apart from the essential nutrients. These compounds are involved in biotic and abiotic stresses response and development, acting as signaling molecules, and in addition, they are related to processes such as photomorphogenesis, nonphotochemical quenching and lipid peroxidation, and attracting pollinators [52].

Brassica vegetables are rich in carotenoids and, among the varieties of *B. oleracea,* kale has the highest levels of lutein and beta-carotene [51]. In Chinese cabbage (*B. rapa* ssp. pekinensis), lutein and β-carotene are mainly distributed in the older leaves and in the flowers, while the zeaxanthin and violaxanthin levels are relatively low [53].

In order for the carotenoid absorption to occur by gut enterocytes, the mechanical and/or enzymatic disruption of the food matrix is necessary. In addition, due to the hydrophobic character of these chemical molecules, the formation of micelles before its absorption is also necessary [54]. Since the carotenoids in fruits and vegetables are present in the chromoplasts, their substructure and the cell wall are the main barriers to the bioavailability of these compounds [55]. Thus, thermal processing as the boiling or the steaming can have positive effects in bioavailability, collaborating to the food matrix disruption, even though negative effects caused by the carotenoids degradation were also reported [56].

The processing methods used in *brassica* vegetables generally increase the carotenoid content [50]. The thermal processing can cause quantitative and qualitative changes by isomerization processes. An increase in the carotenoid content in *brassica* vegetables, such as broccoli, Brussels sprouts, cabbage, cauliflower, and watercress, after boiling and steaming, were reported in many studies [33, 50]. The increase in the total carotenoid content after thermal treatments can also be explained by changes in the cell wall, due to the cellulose degradation, improving the extraction of these compounds, as a result of the denaturation of carotenoids/protein complexes caused after the thermal processing [57]. However, high temperatures can lead to isomerization processes, decreasing the food nutritional values. β-carotene and lutein degradation for the formation of cis-isomer (4–40%) during the thermal processing was described in some studies with *brassica* vegetables (e.g., broccoli and kale) [58]. Thus, a higher retention of cis-isomers was registered in *brassica* vegetables thermally processed in comparison to trans-isomers, leading to losses in the vitamin A content in these foods.

4. Conclusion

Brassica vegetables have attracted increasing attention due to the presence of phytochemicals with beneficial recognized functions to the human organism, reducing the risk of diseases. Variations in the agronomic conditions (e.g., vegetal species, cultivars, development stages, plant organs, fertilization, soil, and pH) and climatic factors (e.g., luminous intensity and water availability) are known for affecting the content and the profile of compounds from the secondary metabolism.

Many studies show that stress can lead to the accumulation of bioactive compounds in plants, generating the production of foods with more benefits to the human health. In contrast, the growth and development are affected, because there is a reallocation of primary metabolites for the formation of secondary metabolites. This reflects in the biomass production and, certainly, in the species production. However, these metabolites, such as GLS, phenolic compounds, and carotenoids, play a fundamental role in the plants' defense against microorganisms, possibly leading to a better adaptation of the plants to the environment and, consequently, to the reduction in the use of agrochemicals. The current knowledge of the climatic factors that affect the content and profile of these phytochemicals in *Brassicaceae* is of scientific and economical interest and can be the base to elaborate strategies for producing plants more resistant to plagues and diseases, reducing the use of agrochemicals and increasing the productivity with a higher nutraceutical potential.

Acknowledgements

The authors gratefully acknowledge the support by São Paulo Research Foundation (FAPESP—Brazil), process 2016/22665-2 and 2016/00972-0, São Paulo State University, and Conselho Nacional de Pesquisa (CNPq e Brazil), process 305177/2015-0.

Conflict of interest

The authors affirm that there is no conflict of interest.

Author details

Cristine Vanz Borges[1], Santino Seabra Junior[2], Franciely S. Ponce[2] and Giuseppina Pace Pereira Lima[1]*

*Address all correspondence to: gpplima@ibb.unesp.br

1 Sao Paulo State University, UNESP, Botucatu, Brazil

2 Department of Agronomy, Mato Grosso State University, Nova Mutum, Brazil

References

[1] Rakow GI. 1 Species Origin and Economic Importance of *Brassica*. In: Berlin HS, editor. *Brassica*. Berlin, Heidelberg; 2004. p. 3-11

[2] Card SD, Hume DE, Roodi D, McGill CR, Millner JP, Johnson RD. Beneficial endophytic microorganisms of *Brassica* - A review. Biological Control. 2015;**90**:102-112

[3] Hafidh RR, Abdulamir AS, Abu Bakar F, Jalilian FA, Jahanshiri F, Abas F, Sekawi Z. Novel anticancer activity and anticancer mechanisms of *Brassica oleracea* L. Var. capitata f. rubra. European Journal of Integrative Medicine. 2013;**5**(5):450-464

[4] Park S, Arasu MV, Jiang N, Choi SH, Lim YP, Park JT, Al-Dhabi NA, Kim SJ. Metabolite profiling of phenolics, anthocyanins and flavonols in cabbage (*Brassica oleracea* var. capitata). Industrial Crops and Products. 2014;**60**:8-14

[5] Forte MBA, Sanctis R, Leonetti G, Manfredelli S, Urbano V. Dietary chemoprevention of colorectal cancer. Annali Italiani di Chirurgia. 2008;**79**(4):261-268

[6] Maria B, Klingen I, Birch ANE, Bones AM, Bruce TJA, Johansen TJ, Meadow R, Mølmann J, Seljåsen R, Smart LE, Stewart D. Phytochemicals of *Brassicaceae* in plant protection and human health - Influences of climate, environment and agronomic practice. Phytochemistry. 2011;**72**(7):538-556

[7] Maynard DN, Hochmuth GJ. Knott's Handbook for Vegetable Growers. 5th ed. New York: John Wiley & Sons; 2006

[8] Bjorkman T, Pearson KJ. High temperature arrest of inflorescence development in broccoli (*Brassica oleracea* var. italica L.). Journal of Experimental Botany. 1998;**49**(318):101-106

[9] Ruelland E, Zachowski A. How plants sense temperature. Environmental and Experimental Botany. 2010;**69**(3):225-232

[10] Lalla JG, Laura VA, Rodrigues APDC, Seabra Júnior S, Silveira DSS, Zago VH, Dornas MF. Competição de cultivares de brócolis tipo cabeça única em Campo Grande. Horticultura Brasileira. 2010;**28**(3):360-363

[11] Thakur BS. Adaptability for yield in some mid-late and late group cauliflower (*Brassica* oleracea var botrytis) genotypes under the mid-hill conditions of Himachal Pradesh. The Indian Journal of Agriculture Sciences. 2017;**76**:37-40

[12] Nespoli A, Cochev JS, Neves SMAS SS. Vegetable Production By Family Agriculture in Alta Floresta, Matogrossense Amazon. CAMPO-TERRITÓRIO Rev. Geogr. agrária. 2015;**10**:159-91

[13] Pereira AA, FMV RE, Fahey KKS, Carvalho R. Influence of temperature and ontogeny on the levels of glucosinolates in broccoli (*Brassica oleracea* Var. Italica) sprouts and their effect on the induction of mammalian phase 2 enzymes. Journal of Agricultural and Food Chemistry. 2002;**50**(21):6239-6244

[14] Ciska E, Martyniak-Przybyszewska B, Kozlowska H. Content of glucosinolates in cruciferous vegetables grown at the same site for two years under different climatic conditions. Journal of Agricultural and Food Chemistry. 2000;**48**(7):2862-2867

[15] Zhang H, Schonhof I, Krumbein A, Gutezeit B, Li L, Stützel H, Schreiner M. Water supply and growing season influence glucosinolate concentration and composition in turnip root (*Brassica rapa* ssp. rapifera L.). Journal of Plant Nutrition and Soil Science. 2008;**171**(2):255-265

[16] Pocasap P, Weerapreeyakul N, Tanthanuch W, Thumanu K. Sulforaphene in *Raphanus sativus* L. var. caudatus Alef increased in late-bolting stage as well as anticancer activity. Asian Pacific Journal of Tropical Biomedicine. 2017;**7**(11):998-1004

[17] Cardenia V, Vivarelli F, Cirillo S, Paolini M, Rodriguez-Estrada MT, Canistro D. Dietary effects of *Raphanus sativus* cv Sango on lipid and oxysterols accumulation in rat brain: A lipidomic study on a non-genetic obesity model. Chemistry and Physics of Lipids. 2017;**207**:206-213

[18] Hubbard TD, Murray IA, Nichols RG, Cassel K, Podolsky M, Kuzu G, Tian Y, Smith P, Kennett MJ, Patterson AD, Perdew GH. Dietary broccoli impacts microbial community structure and attenuates chemically induced colitis in mice in an Ah receptor dependent manner. Journal of Functional Foods. 2017;**37**:685-698

[19] Tong T, Niu YH, Yue Y, chan Wu S, Ding H. Beneficial effects of anthocyanins from red cabbage (*Brassica oleracea* L. var. capitata L.) administration to prevent irinotecan-induced mucositis. Journal of Functional Foods. 2017;**32**:9-17

[20] Jia X, Zhong L, Song Y, Hu Y, Wang G, Sun S. Consumption of citrus and cruciferous vegetables with incident type 2 diabetes mellitus based on a meta-analysis of prospective study. Primary Care Diabetes. 2016;**10**(4):272-280

[21] Traka MH. Health benefits of glucosinolates. Advances in Botanical Research. 2016;**80**:247-279

[22] Dekić MS, Radulović NS, Stojanović NM, Randjelović PJ, Stojanović-Radić ZZ, Najman S, Stojanović S. Spasmolytic, antimicrobial and cytotoxic activities of 5-phenylpentyl isothiocyanate, a new glucosinolate autolysis product from horseradish (*Armoracia rusticana* P. Gaertn., B. Mey. & Scherb., *Brassicaceae*). Food Chemistry. 2017;**232**:329-339

[23] Hassini I, Martinez-Ballesta MC, Boughanmi N, Moreno DA, Carvajal M. Improvement of broccoli sprouts (*Brassica oleracea* L. var. italica) growth and quality by KCl seed priming and methyl jasmonate under salinity stress. Scientia Horticulturae (Amsterdam). 2017;**226**(May):141-151

[24] Hanschen FS, Lamy E, Schreiner M, Rohn S. Reactivity and stability of glucosinolates and their breakdown products in foods. Angewandte Chemie International Edition. 2014;**53**(43):11430-11450

[25] Yi GE, Robin AHK, Yang K, Park JI, Hwang BH, Nou IS. Exogenous methyl jasmonate and salicylic acid induce subspecies-specific patterns of glucosinolate accumulation and gene expression in *Brassica oleracea* L. Molecules. 2016;**21**(10)

[26] Verkerk R, Schreiner M, Krumbein A, Ciska E, Holst B, Rowland I, de Schrijver R, Hansen M, Gerhäuser C, Mithen R, Dekker M. Glucosinolates in *Brassica* vegetables: The influence of the food supply chain on intake, bioavailability and human health. Molecular Nutrition & Food Research. 2009;**53**(Suppl. 2):219-265

[27] Vicas SI, Teusdea AC, Carbunar M, Socaci SA, Socaciu C. Glucosinolates profile and antioxidant capacity of Romanian *Brassica* vegetables obtained by organic and conventional agricultural practices. Plant Foods for Human Nutrition. 2013;**68**(3):313-321

[28] Shapiro TA, Fahey JW, Wade KL, Stephenson KK, Talalay P. Chemoprotective glucosinolates and isothiocyanates of broccoli sprouts: Metabolism and excretion in humans. Cancer Epidemiology, Biomarkers & Prevention. 2001;**10**(5):501-508

[29] Fahey JW, Zhang Y, Talalay P. Broccoli sprouts: An exceptionally rich source of inducers of enzymes that protect against chemical carcinogens. Proceedings of the National Academy of Sciences. 1997;**94**(19):10367-10372

[30] Zanichelli F, Capasso S, Di Bernardo G, Cipollaro M, Pagnotta E, Cartenì M, Casale F, Iori R, Giordano A, Galderisi U. Low concentrations of isothiocyanates protect mesenchymal stem cells from oxidative injuries, while high concentrations exacerbate DNA damage. Apoptosis. 2012;**17**(9):964-974

[31] Wiesner M, Hanschen FS, Schreiner M, Glatt H, Zrenner R. Induced production of 1-methoxy-indol-3-ylmethyl glucosinolate by jasmonic acid and methyl jasmonate in sprouts and leaves of pak choi (*Brassica* rapa ssp. chinensis). International Journal of Molecular Sciences. 2013;**14**(7):14996-15016

[32] Martínez-Ballesta M d C, Moreno DA, Carvajal M. The physiological importance of glucosinolates on plant response to abiotic stress in *Brassica*. International Journal of Molecular Sciences. 2013;**14**(6):11607-11625

[33] Kopsell DA, Sams CE. Increases in shoot tissue pigments, glucosinolates, and mineral elements in sprouting broccoli after exposure to short-duration blue light from light emitting diodes. Journal of the American Society for Horticultural Science. 2013;**138**(1):31-37

[34] Chun JH, Kim S, Arasu MV, Al-Dhabi NA, Chung DY, Kim SJ. Combined effect of nitrogen, phosphorus and potassium fertilizers on the contents of glucosinolates in rocket salad (Eruca sativa Mill.). Saudi Journal of Biological Sciences. 2017;**24**(2):436-443

[35] Augustine R, Bisht NC. Biotic elicitors and mechanical damage modulate Glucosinolate accumulation by co-ordinated interplay of glucosinolate biosynthesis regulators in polyploid *Brassica juncea*. Phytochemistry. 2015;**117**(1):43-50

[36] Bodnaryk RP. Potent effect of jasmonates on indole glucosinolates in oilseed rape and mustard. Phytochemistry. 1994;**35**(2):301-305

[37] Ludwig-Müller J, Schubert B, Pieper K, Ihmig S, Hilgenberg W. Glucosinolate content in susceptible and resistant Chinese cabbage varieties during development of clubroot disease. Phytochemistry. 1997;**44**(3):407-414

[38] Thiruvengadam M, Chung IM. Selenium, putrescine, and cadmium influence health-promoting phytochemicals and molecular-level effects on turnip (*Brassica rapa* ssp. rapa). Food Chemistry. 2015;**173**:185-193

[39] Çiçek N, Çakirlar H. The effect of salinity on some physiological. Bulgarian Journal of Plant Physiology. 2002;**28**(1-2):66-74

[40] Francisco M, Moreno DA, Elena M, Ferreres F, García-viguera C, Velasco P. Simultaneous identification of glucosinolates and phenolic compounds in a representative collection of vegetable *Brassica rapa*. 2009;**1216**:6611-6619

[41] Hanschen FS, Kaufmann M, Kupke F, Hackl T, Kroh LW, Rohn S, Schreiner M. *Brassica* vegetables as sources of epithionitriles: Novel secondary products formed during cooking. Food Chemistry. 2017;**245**(October):564-569

[42] Grubb CD, Abel S. Glucosinolate metabolism and its control. Trends in Plant Science. 2006;**11**(2):89-100

[43] Harborne JB, Baxter H, Moss GP. Phytochemical Dictionary: A Handbook of Bioactive Compounds from Plants. 2nd ed. London: Taylor & Francis; 1999

[44] Verma N, Shukla S. Impact of various factors responsible for fluctuation in plant secondary metabolites. Journal of Applied Research on Medicinal and Aromatic Plants. 2015;**2**:105-113

[45] Singh J, Upadhyay AK, Prasad K, Bahadur A, Rai M. Variability of carotenes, vitamin C, E and phenolics in *Brassica* vegetables. Journal of Food Composition and Analysis. 2007;**20**(2):106-112

[46] Pérez-Gregorio MR, Regueiro J, González-Barreiro C, Rial-Otero R, Simal-Gándara J. Changes in antioxidant flavonoids during freeze-drying of red onions and subsequent storage. Food Control. 2011;**22**(7):1108-1113

[47] Pérez-Balibrea S, Moreno DA, García-Viguera C. Improving the phytochemical composition of broccoli sprouts by elicitation. Food Chemistry. 2011;**129**(1):35-44

[48] Palermo M, Pellegrini N, Fogliano V. The effect of cooking on the phytochemical content of vegetables. Journal of the Science of Food and Agriculture. 2014;**94**(6):1057-1070

[49] Gliszczyńska-Swigło A, Ciska E, Pawlak-Lemańska K, Chmielewski J, Borkowski T, Tyrakowska B. Changes in the content of health-promoting compounds and antioxidant activity of broccoli after domestic processing. Food Additives & Contaminants., vol. 23, no. 11, pp. 1088-1098, 2006.

[50] Giallourou N, Oruna-Concha MJ, Harbourne N. Effects of domestic processing methods on the phytochemical content of watercress (*Nasturtium officinale*). Food Chemistry. 2016;**212**:411-419

[51] Kopsell DA, Kopsell DE, Lefsrud MG, Curran-Celentano J, Dukach LE. Variation in lutein, β-carotene, and chlorophyll concentrations among *Brassica oleracea* cultigens and seasons. Hortscience. 2004;**39**(2):361-364

[52] Farré G, Sanahuja G, Naqvi S, Bai C, Capell T, Zhu C, Christou P. Travel advice on the road to carotenoids in plants. Plant Science. 2010;**179**(1-2):28-48

[53] Baek KJ, SA JY, Lim SH, Park SU. Metabolic profiling in Chinese cabbage (*Brassica rapa* L. subsp. pekinensis) cultivars reveals that glucosinolate content is correlated with carotenoid content. Journal of Agricultural and Food Chemistry. 2016;**64**(21):4426-4434

[54] Sy C, Gleize B, Dangles O, Landrier JF, Veyrat CC, Borel P. Effects of physicochemical properties of carotenoids on their bioaccessibility, intestinal cell uptake, and blood and tissue concentrations. Molecular Nutrition & Food Research. 2012;**56**(9):1385-1397

[55] Kaulmann A, André CM, Schneider YJ, Hoffmann L, Bohn T. Carotenoid and polyphenol bioaccessibility and cellular uptake from plum and cabbage varieties. Food Chemistry. 2016;**197**:325-332

[56] Palmero P, Panozzo A, Simatupang D, Hendrickx M, Van Loey A. Lycopene and β-carotene transfer to oil and micellar phases during in vitro digestion of tomato and red carrot based-fractions. Food Research International. 2014;**64**:831-838

[57] Khachik F, Beecher GR, Goli MB, Lusby WR. Separation, identification, and quantification of carotenoids in fruits, vegetables and human plasma by high performance liquid chromatography. Pure and Applied Chemistry. 1991;**63**(1):71-80

[58] Colle IJP, Lemmens L, Knockaert G, Van Loey A, Hendrickx M. Carotene degradation and isomerization during thermal processing: A review on the kinetic aspects. Critical Reviews in Food Science and Nutrition. 2016;**56**(11):1844-1855

[59] Finley. Proposed criteria for assessing the efficacy of cancer reduction by plant foods enriched in carotenoids, glucosinolates, polyphenols and selenocompounds. Annals of Botany. 2005;**95**:1075-1096

[60] Schonhof I, Blankenburg D, Müller S, Krumbein A. Sulfur and nitrogen supply influence growth, product appearance, and glucosinolate concentration of broccoli. Journal of Soil Science and Plant Nutrition. 2007;**170**:65-72

[61] Charron CS, Sams CE. Glucosinolate Content and Myrosinase Activity in Rapid-cycling *Brassica* oleracea Grown in a Controlled Environment. Journal of the American Society for Horticultural Science. [Internet]. 2004;**129**:321-330

[62] Flaishman MA, Peles Y, Dahan Y, Milo-Cochavi S, Frieman A, Naor A. Differential response of cell-cycle and cell-expansion regulators to heat stress in apple (Malus domestica) fruitlets. Plant Science. [Internet]. Elsevier Ireland Ltd; 2015;**233**:82-94

[63] Makus DJ, Lester G, N TL, Dec LW, N TL, Long W. Effect of soil type, Light intensity, and Cultivar on leaf nutrients in mustard greens. 2002;23-28

[64] Maggio A, De Pascale S, Ruggiero C, Barbieri G. Physiological response of field-grown cabbage to salinity and drought stress. European Journal of Agronomy. 2005;**23**:57-67

[65] Pathirana I, Thavarajah P, Siva N, Wickramasinghe ANK, Smith P, Thavarajah D. Moisture deficit effects on kale (*Brassica* oleracea L. var. acephala) biomass, mineral, and low molecular weight carbohydrate concentrations. Scientia Horticulturae. [Internet]. Amsterdam: Elsevier; 2017;**226**:216-222

[66] Khan MAM, Ulrichs C, Mewis I. Influence of water stress on the glucosinolate profile of *Brassica* oleracea var. italica and the performance of Brevicoryne *brassicae* and Myzus persicae. Entomologia Experimentalis et Applicata. 2010;**137**:229-336

[67] Issarakraisila M, Ma Q, Turner DW. Photosynthetic and growth responses of juvenile Chinese kale (*Brassica* oleracea var. alboglabra) and Caisin (*Brassica* rapa subsp. parachinensis) to waterlogging and water deficit. Scientia Horticulturae. (Amsterdam). 2007;**111**:107-113

[68] López-Berenguer C, García-Viguera C, Carvajal M. Are root hydraulic conductivity responses to salinity controlled by aquaporins in broccoli plants? Plant Soil. 2006;**279**:13-23

[69] López-Berenguer C, Martínez-Ballesta MDC, Moreno DA, Carvajal M, García-Viguera C. Growing hardier crops for better health: Salinity tolerance and the nutritional value of broccoli. Journal of Agricultural and Food Chemistry. 2009;**57**:572-578

[70] Jensen CR, Mogensen VO, Mortensen G, Fieldsend JK, Milford GFJ, Andersen MN, et al. Seed glucosinolate, oil and protein contents of field-grown rape (*Brassica* napus L.) affected by soil drying and evaporative demand. Field Crops Research. 1996;**47**:93-105

[71] Anjana SU, Muhammad I. Agronomy for sustainable development. Ital. Journal of Agronomy. 2008;**3**:77-78

[72] Grattan SR, Grieve CM. Salinity-mineral nutrient relations in horticultural crops. Amsterdam: Journal of Agronomy. 1998;**78**:127-157

[73] Marino D, Ariz I, Lasa B, Santamaría E, Fernández-Irigoyen J, González-Murua C, et al. Quantitative proteomics reveals the importance of nitrogen source to control glucosinolate metabolism in Arabidopsis thaliana and *Brassica* oleracea. Journal of Experimental Botany. 2016;**67**:3313-3323

[74] De Pascale S, Maggio A, Pernice R, Fogliano V, Barbieri G. Sulphur fertilization may improve the nutritional value of *Brassica* rapa L. subsp. sylvestris. European Journal of Agronomy. 2007;**26**:418-424

[75] Li S, Schonhof I, Krumbein A, Li L, Stützel H, Schreiner M. Glucosinolate Concentration in Turnip (*Brassica* rapa ssp. rapifera L.) Roots as Affected by Nitrogen and Sulfur Supply. European Journal of Agronomy. [Internet]. 2007;**55**:8452-8457

Chapter 6

Genetic and Epigenetic Regulation of Vernalization in Brassicaceae

Ayasha Akter, Namiko Nishida, Satoko Takada,
Etsuko Itabashi, Kenji Osabe, Daniel J. Shea and
Ryo Fujimoto

Additional information is available at the end of the chapter

http://dx.doi.org/10.5772/intechopen.74573

Abstract

A wide variation of morphological traits exists in *Brassica rapa* L. and *Brassica oleracea* L., and cultivated vegetable varieties of these species are consumed worldwide. Flowering time is an important agronomic trait in these species and varies among varieties or cultivars. Especially, leafy vegetable species need a high bolting resistance. Isolation of *FLOWERING LOCUS C* (*FLC*), one of the key genes involved in vernalization, has now provided an insight into the molecular mechanism involved in the regulation of flowering time, including the role of histone modification. In the model plant *Arabidopsis thaliana*, *FLC* plays an important role in modulating flowering time. The response to vernalization causes an increase in histone H3 lysine 27 tri-methylation (H3K27me3) that leads to reduced expression of the *FLC* gene. *B. rapa* and *B. oleracea* both contain several paralogs of *FLC* at syntenic regions identified as major flowering time and vernalization response quantitative trait loci (QTL). We introduce the recent research, not only in *A. thaliana*, but also in the genus *Brassica* from a genetic and epigenetic view point.

Keywords: vernalization, flowering time, FLOWERING LOCUS C, histone modification, high bolting resistance

1. Introduction

During the life cycle of plants, the change from vegetative to reproductive growth is a major developmental transition in angiosperms. Flowering is the process where a transformation of the vegetative stem primordia into floral primordia occurs due to biochemical changes. In most plants, once the transition from vegetative to reproductive growth begins, it cannot be reversed. Thus, the proper timing of this transition is advantageous to ensure the successful propagation of offspring. Internal (endogenous cues) and external (environmental stimuli) factors both play important roles in flowering time. As plants are sessile organisms, plants are greatly affected by environmental conditions such as day length (photoperiodism) and temperature. Photoperiodism is controlled via the photoreceptor proteins phytochrome and/or cryptochrome, responsible for sensing red/far-red and blue light, respectively [1]. We typically refer to photoperiod requirements as either long day (LD) or short day (SD) with respect to the length of time that a plant receives daylight. As this photoperiod signal is also tied to the annual cyclical seasonal changes, LD, coinciding with the spring and summer seasons, and SD, associated with the autumn and winter seasons, both play roles in the floral development of several plant species [2]. The regulation of flowering to changes in temperature is known as vernalization. Vernalization is the process that accelerates flowering in response to the prolonged cold winter. Many plants have a vernalization requirement and will actively repress flowering until after an exposure to prolonged cold. This acts to synchronize seed production with the favorable environmental conditions of spring. The presence of certain photoperiods and ambient temperatures after vernalization are also important [3, 4].

Brassica is a genus in the family of Brassicaceae and includes 37 species of flowering plants. Many of these are important both economically and as agricultural crops, with members such as broccoli, brown mustard, brussels sprouts, cabbage, cauliflower, Chinese cabbage, kale, kohlrabi, rape, rutabaga, and turnip. The crops from this genus are sometimes known as cole crops. Three members of the genus *Brassica*: *Brassica rapa*, *Brassica nigra*, and *Brassica oleracea* are denoted as the A, B, and C genomes, respectively. These three species share a unique genomic relationship known as the "Triangle of U" [5]. Allotetraploids between these three species contain two complete diploid genomes derived from the two different parental species, one diploid genome from each parent. The agriculturally important allotetraploid *Brassica napus* (canola or rapeseed) is derived from the interspecific hybridization of the A and C genomes of *B. rapa* and *B. oleracea*, respectively. With the advent of genomic sequencing, the genetic relationship between three diploid species such as *B. rapa*, *B. nigra*, and *B. oleracea*, in the *Brassica* genus has been elucidated further, revealing that they are descended from a common hexaploid ancestor that underwent a whole genome triplication event roughly 15.9 million years ago (MYA), with speciation divergence occurring approximately 4.6 MYA [6].

Different cultivated varieties of the diploid species of *B. rapa* exhibit extreme developmental and morphological diversity, and from the organs consumed they are generally divided into leafy, turnip, and oil types. *B. rapa* crops are normally grown in two seasons, autumn and spring, and their flowering habits are generally controlled by day length and/or temperature. *B. rapa* is a facultative LD plant. Although LD photoperiod conditions accelerate its flowering, it can also flower under SD photoperiod conditions [7]. *B. rapa* is a leafy vegetable, and flowering time is an important developmental trait because bolting can occur before plants reach the harvest stage. Examples include Chinese cabbage and pak choi, where early bolting markedly impairs the product value. Early bolting mostly occurs due to low temperatures at the beginning of cultivation and the longer day lengths during the growing period of the spring season. Thus, the genetic dissection of flowering time control is central to the breeding of late bolting leafy *B. rapa* cultivars. *B. oleracea* (cabbage), a plant-vernalization-responsive species, has become established as one of the most valuable vegetable crops in the Brassicaceae family and is widely consumed by both humans and livestock [8, 9]. Vernalization can be classified into two types: seed-vernalization-responsive and plant-vernalization-responsive, according to the age at which the plant vernalizes in response to low temperature [9]. In the plant-vernalization-responsive type, biennial plants grow vegetatively in the first year and flower in the following year after winter. The vernalization of cabbage normally requires low temperatures of approximately 6–8 weeks in duration that is initiated at the stage of seven to nine leaves, or when the stem diameter reaches 6 mm for the initiation of flowering [8, 9]. The differences in the mechanisms involved in vernalization and flowering between seed- and plant-vernalization-responsive types is of agronomic and scientific interest to understand. As such, attempts have been made to transfer the seed-vernalization character from Chinese cabbage (*B. rapa*) into cabbage (*B. oleracea*) [10], and the plant-vernalization character from cabbage into Chinese cabbage [11]. *B. napus* is an important oilseed crop in the temperate regions of the world. The production of seed in canola depends upon flowering time, thus the adaptation of flowering time is important for breeding. In *B. napus*, the natural variation in flowering time in response to vernalization was characterized into three groups: spring type, winter type, and semi-winter type [12].

Understanding the molecular mechanism(s) responsible for vernalization in the control of flowering is important for the breeding of high bolting resistance in *B. rapa* and *B. oleracea* leafy vegetables. Recent studies on vernalization using *Arabidopsis thaliana*, one of the model organisms used for studying plant biology and the first plant to have its entire genome sequenced, provided key insight into the molecular mechanism of vernalization. The knowledge derived from *A. thaliana* research has been useful for understanding the molecular mechanism of vernalization in the genus *Brassica*. In this chapter, we describe the latest research findings on vernalization in *A. thaliana* and the *Brassica* genus, especially leafy vegetables such as Chinese cabbage (*B. rapa*) and cabbage (*B. oleracea*) with a high bolting resistance.

2. Vernalization research in model plant *Arabidopsis thaliana*

A. thaliana is a small dicotyledonous species used as a model organism for studying plant biology belonging to the family Brassicaceae. In *A. thaliana*, over 180 genes are implicated in flowering time control and these genes are categorized into six major pathways that control flowering time, including the photoperiod/circadian clock pathway, vernalization pathway, ambient temperature pathway, age pathway, autonomous pathway, and gibberellin pathway [13, 14]. It is a much-studied model for vernalization and the transition to the reproductive phase of *A. thaliana* occurs by two related events, the floral transition (initiation of the first flower) and the bolting transition (elongation of the first internode) [15]. Brassicaceae includes many perennial species such as *Arabis alpina* and *Arabidopsis halleri*, and the respective *A. thaliana* orthologous gene is key regulator of flowering transition with seasonal gene expression [16, 17]. In this section, we introduce research on vernalization in *A. thaliana*.

2.1. Genes involved in vernalization

Two key genes, *FRIGIDA* (*FRI*) and *FLOWERING LOCUS C* (*FLC*), have been identified by map-based cloning of naturally occurring early flowering accessions of *A. thaliana*. Rapid cycling accessions have mutations in *FRI*, and loss-of-function mutations have originated independently [3, 18]. The functional *FRI* gene acts upstream of the *FLC* expression within the vernalization pathway. FRI acts as a scaffold protein interacting with FRIGIDA LIKE 1 (FRL1), FRIGIDA ESSENTIAL 1 (FES1), SUPPRESSOR OF FRIGIDA 4 (SUF4), and FLC EXPRESSOR (FLX). These proteins assemble to form a large protein complex, FRIGIDA-containing complex (FRI-C), with SUF4 directly binding to the *FLC* promoter and FRI-C activating *FLC* expression [19].

The *FLC* gene is a floral repressor that contains a MADS box transcriptional regulator protein domain, and maintains a plant's vegetative growth until exposure to prolonged cold is experienced. Within the vegetative apical meristem, FLC interacts with several important genes during vegetative growth by inhibiting the activation of a set of genes required for the transition of the apical meristem to inflorescence, ultimately determining the plant's reproductive fate [20–22]. At the molecular level, FLC blocks flowering by binding to genes that promote flowering and repressing their transcription. Initially, three flowering time genes, *FLOWERING LOCUS T* (*FT*), *SUPPRESSOR OF OVEREXPRESSSON OF CONSTANS 1* (*SOC1*), and *FLOWERING LOCUS D* (*FD*) were reported to be targeted by FLC, with FLC binding to the promoters of *SOC1* and *FD* and to the first intron of *FT* [23, 24]. Later, using antiserum raised against the FLC protein without the conserved MADS domain, more putative *FLC* targeted genes were identified at the whole genome level by chromatin immunoprecipitation sequencing (ChIP-seq). About 500 *FLC* binding sites, mostly located in the promoter region of genes containing one CArG box (the known target of MADS-box proteins) were identified [25]. Two genes (*FT* and *SOC1*) that function downstream of the flowering activator CONSTANS (CO) in the photoperiod pathway were identified as being negatively regulated by *FLC* [4, 14].

In addition to the previously mentioned *FRI*-dependent pathway, the autonomous pathway is also known to repress *FLC* expression. In the autonomous pathway, key genes such as *FCA*, *FLD*, *FLOWERING LATE KH DOMAIN* (*FLK*), *FPA*, *FVE*, *FY*, and *LUMINIDEPENDENS* (*LD*) were identified [4, 22, 26], and mutation in these genes results in the activation of *FLC* and a late flowering phenotype. Thus, *FRI* and the autonomous pathway are internal regulators of basal *FLC* expression via constitutive activation and repression, respectively.

Examination of the regulation of *FLC* by the vernalization pathway in various vernalization-responsive accessions and flowering time mutants of *A. thaliana* showed that the levels of *FLC* mRNA and protein correlated well with flowering time in response to cold treatment [3, 4, 22]. To identify the genes involved in the vernalization pathway, mutants that do not respond to vernalization were characterized. Two mutants termed *vernalization 1* (*vrn1*) and *vrn2* were identified [3, 27, 28]. Cold treatment reduced the *FLC* expression levels in *vrn1 fca-1* or *vrn2 fca-1* double mutants. However, when plants are returned to a warm environment, the suppression of *FLC* expression was not maintained. This suggests that VRN1 and VRN2 are involved in the maintenance of *FLC* repression by vernalization, but not in the initial repression [27, 28]. *VRN1* encodes a nuclear protein with B3 domains, a highly conserved plant-specific transcription factor that binds to DNA [28]. *VRN2* encodes a nuclear-localized zinc-finger protein showing a similarity to Polycomb Group (PcG) proteins of plants and animals [27]. The expression levels of *VRN1* and *VRN2* are not changed by vernalization. However, a third gene involved in the repression of *FLC* by vernalization, *VERNALIZATION INSENSITIVE 3* (*VIN3*), is activated by vernalization, and *VIN3* encodes a plant homeodomain (PHD) finger containing protein [29].

2.2. Epigenetic regulation of *FLC* gene

Epigenetic regulation is defined as changes in gene activities that are inherited through cell divisions without alteration in the DNA sequence. Epigenetic regulation is crucial for the development and adaptation of plants to the changing environment [30, 31]. DNA methylation and histone modification are the best examples of epigenetic modifications. The fundamental subunit of chromatin is the nucleosome, and the nucleosome consists of 147 base pairs of DNA wrapped around an octamer of histone proteins comprised of two tetramers. Each of the two tetramers contains one of each of the core histone proteins H2A, H2B, H3, and H4. The alteration of chromatin structure, which causes changes in transcription, is regulated by various post-translational modifications such as methylation or acetylation of the N-terminal regions of the histone proteins [32]. Histone lysine residues can be mono-, di-, or tri-methylated, and each methylation state is associated with different functions [32]. In plants, histone deacetylation, H3K9me2, and H3K27me3 are associated with gene repression, and histone acetylation, H3K4me3, and H3K36me3 are associated with gene activation [22, 31, 33, 34].

The vernalization response is one example of epigenetic regulation, and *FLC* expression is regulated by chromatin modification [34, 35]. *FLC* is expressed before prolonged cold exposure, and H3K4me3 or H3K36me3 is associated with activation of *FLC* expression [36]. FRI-C facilitates recruitment of chromatin-modifying factors to *FLC*, such as the chromatin remodeling SWR1 complex (delivering H2A.Z variant) or the histone methyltransferases EARLY FLOWERING IN SHORT DAYS (EFS) (a homolog of SET2 that catalyzes H3K36me3) [19], ARABIDOPSIS TRITHORAX LIKE 1 (ATX1) (which catalyzes H3K4me3) [37], and ARABIDOPSIS TRITHORAX-RELATED 7 (ATXR7) [38]. H3K4me3 activity is also mediated by the yeast RNA polymerase II (Pol II) Associated Factor 1 (PAF1) complex, histone H3K4 methyltransferases such as ATX1, ATX2, and ATXR7, and the complex protein associated with Set 1 (COMPASS)-like complex that contains WDR5 HOMOLOG A (WDR5a), EFS, and ARABIDOPSIS Ash2 RELATIVE (ASH2R) [22, 39].

Prolonged cold exposure induces VIN3, a PHD-finger protein, which acts to establish the initial repression of *FLC* [29]. PHD-finger proteins VIN3, VRN5, VIN3/VRN5-like 1 (VEL1) interact with VRN2 protein and form POLYCOMB REPRESSIVE COMPLEX2 (PHD-PRC2) complex [29, 40, 41]. *FLC* repression by vernalization is associated with the enrichment of H3K27me3, which is mediated by the PHD-PRC2 mechanism [41]. During prolonged cold exposure, H3K27me3 is enriched in chromatin at the *FLC* transcription/translation start sites [42]. After cold exposure, during growth at higher temperatures, the H3K27me3 modification extends across the *FLC* gene [42]. The initial transcriptional repression of *FLC* is PRC2-independent, but the stable maintenance of repression requires PRC2 [27]. The maintenance of *FLC* silencing under warm conditions after cold exposure is therefore mediated by PHD-PRC2 spreading H3K27me3 over the *FLC* locus. In addition, LIKE HETEROCHROMATIN PROTEIN 1 (LHP1), which is associated with H3K27me3, and VRN1 are required for the maintenance of stable *FLC* repression [28, 43, 44].

FLC is epigenetically silenced by vernalization, but *FLC* needs to be reactivated to restore the requirement for vernalization in each subsequent generation. *FLC* expression is repressed in gametogenesis, regardless of the parental state of vernalization, and its expression increases as the embryo develops [45, 46]. Some autonomous pathway genes, which upregulate *FLC* in vegetative tissues, are required for *FLC* expression in the early embryo [46]. In contrast, *FRI* and *SUF4* are not required to reset the expression of *FLC*, however, they are required to maintain it after reactivation of *FLC* [46]. EARLY FLOWERING 6 (ELF6) is a jumonji domain H3K27me3 demethylase protein and is expressed at high levels in both flowers and embryos, but at low levels in seedlings [47]. Resetting of the vernalized state at the *FLC* locus in the next generation requires H3K27 demethylation by ELF6 [47]. However, *FLC* expression in some non-vernalized *elf6* mutants was found to be lower than in non-vernalized wild type, but the expression level was fully restored in the next generation [48]. Thus, there may be another factor associated with the resetting of *FLC* expression. LEAFY COTYLEDON1 (LEC1) encodes a seed-specific NF-YB transcription factor that is a subunit of NF-Y that binds to NF-C and NF-A, and regulates embryogenesis. LEC1 NF-Y engages EFS, which is associated with H3K36me3, and the SWR1 complex, remodeling the chromatin state at the *FLC* locus to a transcriptionally active euchromatic state during embryogenesis [46, 48]. This activity suggests that LEC1 NF-Y binds to the *FLC* promoter, displacing Polycomb proteins and recruiting EFS, and that the maintenance of a euchromatic state at the *FLC* locus by LEC1 inhibits the transmission of repressive chromatin marks [48].

2.3. Long noncoding RNA induced by cold treatments in the *FLC* locus

Advanced technologies such as tiling arrays or RNA-sequencing (RNA-seq), use high-throughput sequencing to enable the discovery of long noncoding transcripts. It has been shown that some long noncoding RNAs (lncRNAs) are involved in the regulation of gene expression through interactions with associated proteins. Several PRC2-associated lncRNAs have been identified in mammals, for example, *XIST* targets PRC2 to the X chromosome or HOTAIR targets PRC2 to the *HOX* gene, resulting in silencing of target genes [22]. Using a custom array covering the 50 kb region around *FLC*, with single-nucleotide resolution of both strands, lncRNAs termed cold-induced long antisense intragenic RNAs (COOLAIR) have been identified. COOLAIR encompasses most of the *FLC* locus, from the 5′ start to the 3′ polyadenylation sites, and COOLAIR is alternatively polyadenylated and spliced. The induction of COOLAIR occurs after 14 days of cold treatment in wild type and *vin3–4* mutants, which is earlier than *VIN3* induction (20 days after transfer to cold), and the suppression of unspliced sense *FLC* transcription was observed before the maximum induction of *VIN3* [29, 49]. COOLAIR promoter-driven antisense transcription of a reporter gene could lead to transient cold-induced repression, suggesting that COOLAIR contributes to the early repression of sense *FLC* transcription transiently before the stable repression that is mediated by the PHD-PRC2 complex [49]. However, plants having T-DNA insertions in the region covering COOLAIR where COOLAIR expression or upregulation of COOLAIR is not observed during cold treatment, showed normal repression of sense *FLC* by vernalization. This suggests that the production of COOLAIR transcripts is not an essential component of vernalization-induced repression of *FLC* [50]. Because of this, while COOLAIR is considered to be involved in the autonomous pathway and the PRC2-mediated epigenetic silencing of *FLC*, its function in the cold-induced silencing of *FLC* is still controversial [50–52]. After the degradation of *FLC* mRNA via COOLAIR, COOLAIR transcription is then reduced by the formation of an RNA-DNA hybrid within its promoter, R-loop [53].

Another lncRNA, COLD ASSISTED INTRONIC NONCODING RNA (COLDAIR), has been identified in the first intron of *FLC* in the sense direction. COLDAIR contains a 5′ cap structure but is not polyadenylated. COLDAIR is induced during cold exposure and reaches its maximum level of expression at around 20 days of cold exposure. The expression level then returns to the pre-vernalized level after more than 30 days of cold. The induction of COLDAIR occurs earlier than *VIN3* induction, but later than the induction of COOLAIR. The transcription start site of COLDAIR is located within the VERNALIZATION RESPONSE ELEMENT (VRE), a region important for the stable repression of *FLC* by vernalization [44]. COLDAIR interacts with *FLC* chromatin and one of the components of the PRC2 complex, CURLY LEAF (CLF), specifically during cold exposure. Reduced COLDAIR by RNA interference showed that *FLC* repression was not maintained when plants were returned to a warm growth condition after vernalization. COLDAIR mutants decrease the association of PRC2 and H3K27me3 accumulation [54]. In addition, the repression of *FLC* expression by cold treatment was not maintained in the COLDAIR mutants once the plants were moved to normal growth conditions [55]. Increased expression of *CLF* and enrichment of H3K27me3 by vernalization were not observed in knockdown lines of COLDAIR, indicating that COLDAIR plays a role in the establishment of the stable maintenance of *FLC* repression during vernalization by recruitment of the PHD-PRC2 complex to *FLC* chromatin [54].

RNA immunoprecipitation (RIP) using the antibody against CLF followed by a tiled RT-PCR identified COLDWRAP (cold of winter-induced noncoding RNA from the promoter) overlapping the promoter region of *FLC*. COLDWRAP associated with PRC2 throughout cold exposure. COLDWRAP transcripts increased during cold exposure, and were maintained even after cold exposure. COLDWRAP has a 5′ cap structure but is not polyadenylated. COLDWRAP is 316 bp in length, and its transcription start site is 225 bp upstream from the *FLC* mRNA transcription start site. COLDWRAP mutants showed an absence of stable repression of *FLC* expression by cold exposure, with a low level of recruitment of PRC2 and H3K27me3 accumulation, suggesting that COLDWRAP is involved in PRC2-mediated *FLC* silencing by vernalization [56].

3. Vernalization research in the genus *Brassica*

Flowering time is very important for the harvest of valuable agricultural products because the flowering that is induced by exposure to cold temperatures, known as bolting, can occur. This is especially the case in vernalization-sensitive leafy vegetables of the genus *Brassica* (*B. rapa* and *B. oleracea*). Because bolting causes the devaluation of agricultural products, a high bolting resistance is of economic significance for cultivar breeding. Additionally, the control of flowering time is also critical for the yield of seeds in canola (*B. napus*) because the appropriate timing of flowering maximizes both seed production and quality. The *FLC* gene maintains a plant's vegetative growth phase until exposure to prolonged cold, and is highly conserved among members of the Brassicaceae family [57], suggesting that the *FLC* gene is an important factor for the breeding of highly bolting resistant cultivars in leafy vegetables. Indeed, previous studies have already supported this possibility. This section introduces the research of flowering in the genus *Brassica,* mainly focusing on the *FLC* gene.

3.1. Species in the genus *Brassica* has the paralogs of *FLC* genes

Recently, the whole genome sequences of the diploid species, *B. rapa*, *B. nigra*, and *B. oleracea*, and the allotetraploid species, *B. napus* and *B. juncea* have been determined. From these genome sequences, it is already known that there are multiple *FLC* paralogs in the genus *Brassica*. Four *FLC* paralogs, Bra009055 (*BrFLC1*), Bra028599 (*BrFLC2*), Bra006051 (*BrFLC3*), and Bra022771 (*BrFLC5*) were found in the reference genome of *B. rapa*, Chiifu-401-42, but Bra022771 is possibly a pseudogene because of the two deleted exons. Two *BoFLC* (Bol008758, Bol043693) paralogs are found in the *B. oleracea* var. *capitata* homozygous line 02–12, while four *BoFLC* paralogs are found in TO1000DH3, a doubled haploid derived from a rapid cycling *B. oleracea*. In the reference genome of allotetraploid species of *B. napus* (AC genome), nine *FLC* paralogs were found in the European winter oilseed cultivar Darmor-bzh with four *FLC*s in the A_n subgenome and five within the C_n subgenome [58].

3.2. QTL controlling flowering time

In the genus *Brassica,* several quantitative trait loci (QTLs) affecting flowering time have been identified. To identify the genes involved in flowering time QTLs, populations derived from parents that show differences for flowering time were used.

In *B. rapa*, several QTLs for flowering time (VFR1, 2, and 3 in non-vernalized condition and FR1, 2, and 3 in vernalized condition) were identified using an F_2 population derived from a cross between an annual and a biennial oil seed cultivars [59, 60]. Later, VFR2 and FR1 were located in the regions covering *BrFLC1* and *BrFLC2*, respectively [61, 62]. Using a multi-population derived from several parental lines (rapid cycling, Chinese cabbage, yellow sarson, pak-choi, and a Japanese vegetable turnip variety) eight QTLs for flowering were detected, and one major QTL co-localized with *BrFLC2* [63]. *BrFLC1* and *BrFLC2* were linked to QTLs that control bolting, budding, and flowering time using an F_2 population derived from an early flowering oilseed rape line, yellow sarson, and a late flowering line of the Japanese commercial komatsuna variety, osome [64]. In yellow sarson, a decrease in *BrFLC2* transcripts was observed and was considered to be due to a nucleotide substitution occurring upstream of the start codon [64]. QTL analyses using other parental combinations between pak-choi and yellow sarson also showed the co-localization of a major QTL with *BrFLC2* [65, 66]. QTL analysis using a recombinant inbred line population produced from a cross between a caixin line (L58, ssp. *parachinensis*) and a yellow sarson line (R-o-18, ssp. *tricolaris*) detected two QTLs in both the spring and autumn seasons, and the *BrFT2* gene is co-localized with a QTL. Later flowering is caused by a transposon insertion in the second intron of *BrFT2*. In another QTL, *BrFLC2* was located, and the earlier flowering line has a 57-bp deletion covering the fourth exon and fifth intron [67]. QTL analyses by different groups over many years have shown that a major QTL of flowering time co-localized with *BrFLC2*. Because of the early flowering line, yellow sarson was used as a parent for making the populations for QTL analysis in all groups, it seems likely that all the groups detected the defects of *BrFLC2* function in yellow sarson as a flowering time QTL. QTL analysis using an F_2 population derived from a cross between an extremely late bolting line (Nou 6 gou, PL6) and early bolting line (A9709) of Chinese cabbage was performed in two different conditions, greenhouse and open field. Five QTLs were detected, but the QTLs did not map to the same position between the two conditions. Three of five QTLs were co-localized with *BrFTa* (greenhouse), *BrFLC1* (open field), and *BrFLC5* (open field) [68]. In another parental combination in Chinese cabbage, an F_2 population was developed from the cross of an early bolting parent of commercial F_1 varieties, Early, and an extremely late bolting breeding line, Tsukena No. 2. In this analysis, the QTLs for bolting time after vernalization co-localized with the late bolting alleles of *BrFLC2* and *BrFLC3*. These two genes carry large insertions in the first intron, suggesting that a weak repression of *BrFLC2* and *BrFLC3* transcripts by vernalization causes the extremely late bolting of Tsukena No. 2 [69]. Furthermore, this group succeeded in developing new F_1 hybrids of Chinese cabbage by introducing these two *FLC* alleles from Tsukena No. 2 [70].

In *B. oleracea*, QTL analysis using a population derived from a DH line of broccoli, Green Comet (var. *italica*), and a DH line of cabbage, Reiho (var. *capitata*), identified a major QTL covering *BoFLC2*, while *BoFLC1*, *BoFLC3*, and *BoFLC5* were not linked to the QTLs [71]. In addition, Green Comet (non-vernalization type) has a single base deletion in exon 4 leading to the frame-shift, suggesting that *BoFLC2* contributes to the control of flowering time [71]. Another group performed QTL analysis using the population derived from a rapid cycling line of *B. oleracea* var. *alboglabra* (A12DHd) and the broccoli variety, Green Duke. Because these two lines contain non-functional copies of *BoFLC2* (named *BoFLC4* in this paper), there is a deletion in the A12DHs, and a single base deletion in exon 4 in Green Duke, it was concluded that *BoFLC2* is not responsible for the flowering time difference between the two lines [72]. Later, the association between flowering time (under both glasshouse and field conditions) and a QTL at *BoFLC2* has been shown using the population derived from two purple sprouting broccoli lines, E5 and E9; E9 requires longer cold periods than E5 to head [73].

QTL analysis was also performed in *B. napus*, and QTLs for flowering time were co-localized with the genes involved in flowering time in *A. thaliana*. Using a population derived from a biennial rapeseed cultivar, Major, and the annual canola cultivar, Stellar, four QTLs (VFN1, 2, 3 in non-vernalized condition and FN1 in vernalized condition) were detected. One major

QTL, VFN1, co-localized with the region collinear with the top of chromosome 4 in *A. thaliana* covering the *FRI* gene [60, 74]. Six *FT* paralogs have been mapped in the *B. napus* genome and three (*BnA2.FT, BnC6.FT.a,* and *BnC6.FT.b*) genes were co-localized with two major QTL clusters for flowering time using populations from the European winter cultivar, Tapidor, and the Chinese semi-winter cultivar, Ningyou 7 [75]. Using the same population, *BnaA.FRI.a* was co-localized to a major flowering time QTL in multiple environments [76]. QTL analyses were performed under field and greenhouse conditions using a population from two Australian *B. napus* cultivars, Skipton and Ag-Spectrum, and the number of QTL detected differed between the two growth conditions. Flowering time genes such as *FLC* were localized within marker intervals associated with flowering time [77, 78]. A total of 158 European winter type *B. napus* inbred lines were genotyped to investigate the association with flowering time, plant height, and seed yield by a genome-wide association study (GWAS). This study revealed that the flowering time regulators, *Bna.FLC* and *Bna.CO,* were absent from the candidate regions associated with flowering time [79]. Another GWAS study examined the flowering times and genome architectures of 188 accessions of *B. napus* collected from different geographic locations around the world, showing associations between flowering time and regions within 20 kb of *FT, FLC,* and *FRI* [12].

3.3. Regulation of *FLC*s by vernalization in the genus *Brassica*

From QTL analyses, it has been demonstrated that multiple *FRI* or *FLC* paralogs are involved in the flowering times of *B. rapa, B. oleracea,* and *B. napus*. The transformation of *BoFRIa* complemented the loss of FRI function in *A. thaliana,* indicating that BoFRI has the same function as AtFRI [80]. In the case of *FLC* paralogs, the early flowering line yellow sarson has a non-functional *BrFLC2* [64, 67], and a naturally occurring splicing mutation in the *BrFLC1* gene is associated with flowering time variation [81]. In *B. oleracea,* an early flowering line of broccoli has a frame-shift mutation in exon 4 of *BoFLC2* [71]. In addition, 40% of flowering time variation in cauliflower (var. *botrytis*) was explained by the same mutation in *BoFLC2* [82]. Furthermore, transgenic plants overexpressing *BnFLC* paralogs in *A. thaliana* showed a late flowering phenotype, indicating that all five *BnFLCs* have similar function to *AtFLC* [83], and three *FLC*s (*BrFLC1, BrFLC 2,* and *BrFLC3*) have been confirmed to be a floral repressor in *B. rapa* [84]. These results indicate that FLC paralogs function as a floral repressor, and play an important role in the vernalization requirement.

In *B. rapa,* it has been shown that there is a difference in the expression levels of the *FLC* paralogs [85]. The coding sequences for the *FLC* paralogs are relatively conserved between *Brassica* species, but the alignment of the upstream sequences or introns are more divergent [57]. This suggests that these differences may account for the different steady state expression levels among *BrFLC* paralogs, or variation of the vernalization requirement.

In *B. rapa* grown under normal conditions, all four *BrFLC* paralogs were expressed in the leaves. The expression of *BrFLC* genes was reduced after vernalization, and the repression was stably maintained after returning to ambient temperatures. Before cold treatment, only *BrFLC1* showed accumulation of both H3K4me3 and H3K36me3 modifications, while three of the *BrFLC* paralogs (*BrFLC2, BrFLC3,* and *BrFLC5*) had only H3K4me3. After 4 weeks of cold treatment, the accumulation of H3K27me3 was observed in *BrFLC1*, *BrFLC2*, and *BrFLC3*, and H3K27me3 was maintained after returning to a warm temperature [85]. These results indicate that, like *A. thaliana*, the repression of *BrFLC* expression by prolonged cold treatment was associated with the states of histone modification. The first intron, the promoter region, and exon 1 are important for *FLC* repression in *A. thaliana* [86], and lncRNA COLDAIR is expressed from the mid-region of the first intron in *A. thaliana* [54, 87]. Although insertions in the first intron cause a weak repression of *BrFLC2* and *BrFLC3* transcripts by vernalization in *B. rapa*, sequence similarity to the VRE in the first intron or to the COLDAIR of *A. thaliana* were not detected in the first intron of any of the *B. rapa* paralogs [69]. At least, COLDAIR-like transcripts in *B. rapa* were not detected. By contrast, COOLAIR-like transcripts were detected only from *BrFLC2*, and these transcripts were induced by cold treatment. The plant growth cycle was shortened by the over-expression of *FLC* natural antisense transcripts (NATs) (COOLAIR-like) resulting in decreased flowering time and *FLC* expression, suggesting that the activity of the *BrFLC2* gene was suppressed by *BrFLC* NATs during cold condition [88]. *BoFLC2* was shown to be a major determinant of heading date variation and vernalization response through allelic variation, and sequence polymorphisms in *BoFLC2* alter the sensitivity and silencing dynamics of its expression [73].

3.4. Perspective of vernalization research in the genus *Brassica*

In leafy vegetables such as Chinese cabbage or cabbage, a high bolting resistance is an important trait for cultivation, indicating that understanding the molecular mechanisms of the vernalization requirement is important for breeding. While research into vernalization and flowering time has provided a wealth of information, a complete understanding of the molecular mechanism controlling the vernalization requirement has not yet been elucidated. In contrast to *A. thaliana*, where histone modifications such as active marks, H3K4me3 and H3K36me3, or repressive marks, H3K9me2 and H3K27me3, have been characterized at the whole genome level by ChIP-seq, such analysis has yet to be conducted in the genus *Brassica*. Comparison of the histone modification states, especially H3K27me3, at the whole genome level between vernalized and non-vernalized plants will identify the genes other than *FLC*s involved in the regulation of vernalization. In addition, combining histone modification data with transcriptome data may facilitate the identification of genes involved in the regulation of vernalization. In *A. thaliana*, it has been revealed that lncRNAs such as COOLAIR, COLDAIR, and COLDWRAP are involved in vernalization [49, 54, 56]. Currently, COOLAIR-like transcripts were detected only from *BrFLC2*, and these transcripts were involved in the suppression of *BrFLC2* and maybe other *BrFLCs* [88]. However, in *B. rapa*, there is no report about the transcripts of COLDAIR or COLDWRAP, and regions sharing sequence similarity to the COLDAIR found in *A. thaliana* were not detected in the first intron of any of the *B. rapa* paralogs [69]. Therefore, there is a possibility that lncRNAs that do not show sequence similarity to COLDAIR or COLDWRAP may be involved in the regulation of repression of *FLC* in the genus *Brassica*. To examine this possibility, lncRNAs whose expression changes in response to vernalization will need to be assessed by RNA-seq. Thus, there exists a need to identify the sequences important for vernalization, termed VREs, within the genus *Brassica*; and to examine any sequence polymorphisms that may exist with respect to the vernalization response. This will help to identify important regions and explicate their relationship to sensitivity of vernalization. If there are any correlations, they will be useful for marker-assisted selection, and serve as important tools for breeding in the genus *Brassica*.

Acknowledgements

This work was supported by Grant-in-Aid for Scientific Research (B) (15H04433) (JSPS) and Hyogo Science and Technology Association.

Conflict of interest

The authors declare that they have no conflict of interest.

Author details

Ayasha Akter[1,2], Namiko Nishida[1], Satoko Takada[1], Etsuko Itabashi[3], Kenji Osabe[4], Daniel J. Shea[5] and Ryo Fujimoto[1]*

*Address all correspondence to: leo@people.kobe-u.ac.jp

1 Graduate School of Agricultural Science, Kobe University, Kobe, Japan

2 Faculty of Agriculture, Bangladesh Agricultural University, Mymensingh, Bangladesh

3 Institute of Vegetable and Floriculture Science, NARO, Tsu, Japan

4 Okinawa Institute of Science and Technology Graduate University, Okinawa, Japan

5 Graduate School of Science and Technology, Niigata University, Niigata, Japan

References

[1] Más P, Devlin PF, Panda S, Kay SA. Functional interaction of phytochrome B and cryptochrome 2. Nature. 2000;**408**:207-211. DOI: 10.1038/35041583

[2] Corbesier L, Coupland G. Photoperiodic flowering of *Arabidopsis*: Integrating genetic and physiological approaches to characterization of the floral stimulus. Plant, Cell & Environment. 2005;**28**:54-66. DOI: 10.1111/j.1365-3040.2005.01283.x

[3] Henderson IR, Dean C. Control of *Arabidopsis* flowering: The chill before the bloom. Development. 2004;**131**:3829-3838. DOI: 10.1242/dev.01294

[4] Kim DH, Doyle MR, Sung S, Amasino RM. Vernalization: Winter and the timing of flowering in plants. Annual Review of Cell and Developmental Biology. 2009;**25**:277-299. DOI: 10.1146/annurev.cellbio.042308.113411

[5] UN: Genome analysis in *Brassica* with special reference to the experimental formation of *B. napus* and peculiar mode of fertilization. Japanese Journal of Botany. 1935;**7**:389-452

[6] Cheng F, Wu J, Wang X. Genome triplication drove the diversification of *Brassica* plants. Horticulture Research. 2014;**1**:14024. DOI: 10.1038/hortres.2014.24

[7] Falik O, Hoffmann I, Novoplansky A. Say it with flowers: Flowering acceleration by root communication. Plant Signaling & Behavior. 2014;**9**:e28258. DOI: 10.4161/psb.28258

[8] Ito H, Saito T, Hatayama T. Time and temperature factors for the flower formation in cabbage II. The site of vernalization and the nature of vernalization sensitivity. Tohoku. Journal of Agricultural Research. 1966;**17**:1-15

[9] Friend DJC. *Brassica*. Harlevy AH, editor. Handbook of Flowering. CRC Press; 1985. pp. 44-77

[10] Hossain MM, Inden H, Asahira T. Seed vernalized interspecific hybrids through in vitro ovule culture in *Brassica*. Plant Science. 1990;**68**:95-102. DOI: 10.1016/0168-9452(90)90157-J

[11] Shea DJ, Tomaru Y, Itabashi E, Nakamura Y, Miyazaki T, Kakizaki T, Naher TN, Shimizu M, Fujimoto R, Fukai E, Okazaki K. The production and characterization of a *BoFLC2* introgressed *Brassica rapa* by repeated backcrossing to an F_1. Breeding Science. 2018 in press

[12] Raman H, Raman R, Coombes N, Song J, Prangnell R, Bandaranayake C, Tahira R, Sundaramoorthi V, Killian A, Meng J, Dennis ES, Balasubramanian S. Genome-wide association analyses reveal complex genetic architecture underlying natural variation for flowering time in canola. Plant, Cell and Environment. 2016;**39**:1228-1239. DOI: 10.1111/pce.12644

[13] Srikanth A, Schmid M. Regulation of flowering time: All roads lead to Rome. Cellular and Molecular Life Sciences. 2011;**68**:2013-2037. DOI: 10.1007/s00018-011-0673-y

[14] Andrés F, Coupland G. The genetic basis of flowering responses to seasonal cues. Nature Reviews Genetics. 2012;**13**:627-639. DOI: 10.1038/nrg3291

[15] Pouteau S, Albertini C. The significance of bolting and floral transitions as indicators of reproductive phase change in *Arabidopsis*. Journal of Experimental Botany. 2009;**60**:3367-3377. DOI: 10.1093/jxb/erp173

[16] Wang R, Farrona S, Vincent C, Joecker A, Schoof H, Turck F, Alonso-Blanco C, Coupland G, Albani MC. *PEP1* regulates perennial flowering in *Arabis alpina*. Nature. 2009;**459**:423-427. DOI: 10.1038/nature07988

[17] Aikawa S, Kobayashi MJ, Satake A, Shimizu KK, Kudoh H. Robust control of the seasonal expression of the *Arabidopsis FLC* gene in a fluctuating environment. Proceedings

of the National Academy of Sciences of the United States of America. 2010;**107**:11632-11637. DOI: 10.1073/pnas.0914293107

[18] Johanson U, West J, Lister C, Michaels S, Amasino R, Dean C. Molecular analysis of *FRIGIDA*, a major determinant of natural variation in *Arabidopsis* flowering time. Science. 2000;**290**:344-347. DOI: 10.1126/science.290.5490.344

[19] Choi K, Kim J, Hwang HJ, Kim SY, Park C, Kim SY, Lee I. The FRIGIDA complex activates transcription of *FLC*, a strong flowering repressor in *Arabidopsis*, by recruiting chromatin modification factors. The Plant Cell. 2011;**23**:289-303. DOI: 10.1105/tpc.110.075911

[20] Michaels SD, Amasino RM. *FLOWERING LOCUS C* encodes a novel MADS domain protein that acts as a repressor of flowering. The Plant Cell. 1999;**11**:949-956. DOI: 10.1105/tpc.11.5.949

[21] Sheldon CC, Burn JE, Perez PP, Metzger J, Edwards JA, Peacock WJ, Dennis ES. The *FLF* MADS box gene: A repressor of flowering in Arabidopsis regulated by vernalization and methylation. The Plant Cell. 1999;**11**:445-458. DOI: 10.1105/tpc.11.3.445

[22] Whittaker C, Dean C. The *FLC* locus: A platform for discoveries in epigenetics and adaptation. Annual Review of Cell and Developmental Biology. 2017;**33**:555-575. DOI: 10.1146/annurev-cellbio-100616-060546

[23] Helliwell CA, Wood CC, Robertson M, Peacock WJ, Dennis ES. The Arabidopsis FLC protein interacts directly *in vivo* with *SOC1* and *FT* chromatin and is part of a high-molecular-weight protein complex. The Plant Journal. 2006;**46**:183-192. DOI: 10.1111/j.1365-313X.2006.02686. x

[24] Searle I, He Y, Turck F, Vincent C, Fornara F, Kröber S, Amasino RA, Coupland G. The transcription factor *FLC* confers a flowering response to vernalization by repressing meristem competence and systemic signaling in *Arabidopsis*. Genes & Development. 2006;**20**:898-912. DOI: 10.1101/gad.373506

[25] Deng W, Ying H, Helliwell CA, Taylor JM, Peacock WJ, Dennis ES. FLOWERING LOCUS C (FLC) regulates development pathways throughout the life cycle of *Arabidopsis*. Proceedings of the National Academy of Sciences of the United States of America. 2011;**108**:6680-6685. DOI: 10.1073/pnas.1103175108

[26] Simpson GG. The autonomous pathway: Epigenetic and post-transcriptional gene regulation in the control of *Arabidopsis* flowering time. Current Opinion in Plant Biology. 2004;7:570-574. DOI: 10.1016/j.pbi.2004.07.002

[27] Gendall AR, Levy YY, Wilson A, Dean C. The *VERNALIZATION 2* gene mediates the epigenetic regulation of vernalization in *Arabidopsis*. Cell. 2001;**107**:525-535. DOI: 10.1016/S0092-8674(01)00573-6

[28] Levy YY, Mesnage S, Mylne JS, Gendall AR, Dean C. Multiple roles of *Arabidopsis VRN1* in vernalization and flowering time control. Science. 2002;**297**:243-246. DOI: 10.1126/science.1072147

[29] Sung S, Amasino RM. Vernalization in *Arabidopsis thaliana* is mediated by the PHD finger protein VIN3. Nature. 2004;**427**:159-164. DOI: 10.1038/nature02195

[30] Richards EJ. Natural epigenetic variation in plant species: A view from the field. Current Opinion in Plant Biology. 2011;**14**:204-209. DOI: 10.1016/j.pbi.2011.03.009

[31] Fujimoto R, Sasaki T, Ishikawa R, Osabe K, Kawanabe T, Dennis ES. Molecular mechanisms of epigenetic variation in plants. International Journal of Molecular Science. 2012;**13**:9900-9922. DOI: 10.3390/ijms13089900

[32] Fuchs J, Demidov D, Houben A, Schubert I. Chromosomal histone modification patterns–from conservation to diversity. Trends in Plant Science. 2006;**11**:199-208. DOI: 10.1016/j.tplants.2006.02.008

[33] Bastow R, Mylne JS, Lister C, Lippman Z, Martienssen RA, Dean C. Vernalization requires epigenetic silencing of *FLC* by histone methylation. Nature. 2004;**427**:164-167. DOI: 10.1038/nature02269

[34] Dennis ES, Peacock WJ. Epigenetic regulation of flowering. Current Opinion in Plant Biology. 2007;**10**:520-527. DOI: 10.1016/j.pbi.2007.06.009

[35] Groszmann M, Greaves IK, Albert N, Fujimoto R, Helliwell CA, Dennis ES, Peacock WJ. Epigenetics in plants-vernalisation and hybrid vigour. Biochimica et Biophysica Acta. 2011;**1809**:427-437. DOI: 10.1016/j.bbagrm.2011.03.006

[36] Ko JH, Mitina I, Tamada Y, Hyun Y, Choi Y, Amasino RM, Noh B, Noh YS. Growth habit determination by the balance of histone methylation activities in *Arabidopsis*. The EMBO Journal. 2010;**29**:3208-3215. DOI: 10.1038/emboj.2010.198

[37] Pien S, Fleury D, Mylne JS, Crevillen P, Inzé D, Avramova Z, Dean C, Grossniklaus U. ARABIDOPSIS TRITHORAX1 dynamically regulates *FLOWERING LOCUS C* activation via histone 3 lysine 4 trimethylation. The Plant Cell. 2008;**20**:580-588. DOI: 10.1105/tpc.108.058172

[38] Berr A, Xu L, Gao J, Cognat V, Steinmetz A, Dong A, Shen WH. *SET DOMAIN GROUP25* encodes a histone methyltransferase and is involved in *FLOWERING LOCUS C* activation and repression of flowering. Plant Physiology. 2009;**151**:1476-1485. DOI: 10.1104/pp.109.143941

[39] He Y, Doyle MR, Amasino RM. PAF1-complex-mediated histone methylation of *FLOWERING LOCUS C* chromatin is required for the vernalization-responsive, winter-annual habit in *Arabidopsis*. Genes & Development. 2004;**18**:2774-2784. DOI: 10.1101/gad.1244504

[40] Wood CC, Robertson M, Tanner G, Peacock WJ, Dennis ES, Helliwell CA. The *Arabidopsis thaliana* vernalization response requires a polycomb-like protein complex that also includes VERNALIZATION INSENSITIVE 3. Proceedings of the National Academy of Sciences of the United States of America. 2006;**103**:14631-14636. DOI: 10.1073/pnas.0606385103

[41] De Lucia F, Crevillen P, Jones AM, Greb T, Dean C. A PHD-polycomb repressive complex 2 triggers the epigenetic silencing of *FLC* during vernalization. Proceedings of the National Academy of Sciences of the United States of America. 2008;**105**:16831-16836. DOI: 10.1073/pnas.0808687105

[42] Finnegan EJ, Dennis ES. Vernalization-induced trimethylation of histone H3 lysine 27 at *FLC* is not maintained in mitotically quiescent cells. Current Biology. 2007;**17**:1978-1983. DOI: 10.1016/j.cub.2007.10.026

[43] Mylne JS, Barrett L, Tessadori F, Mesnage S, Johnson L, Bernatavichute YV, Jacobsen SE, Fransz P, Dean C. LHP1, the *Arabidopsis* homologue of HETEROCHROMATIN PROTEIN1, is required for epigenetic silencing of *FLC*. Proceedings of the National Academy of Sciences of the United States of America. 2006;**103**:5012-5017. DOI: 10.1073/pnas.0507427103

[44] Sung S, He Y, Eshoo TW, Tamada Y, Johnson L, Nakahigashi K, Goto K, Jacobsen SE, Amasino RM. Epigenetic maintenance of the vernalized state in *Arabidopsis thaliana* requires LIKE HETEROCHROMATIN PROTEIN 1. Nature Genetics. 2006;**38**:706-710. DOI: 10.1038/ng1795

[45] Sheldon CC, Hills MJ, Lister C, Dean C, Dennis ES, Peacock WJ. Resetting of *FLOWERING LOCUS C* expression after epigenetic repression by vernalization. Proceedings of the National Academy of Sciences of the United States of America. 2008;**105**:2214-2219. DOI: 10.1073/pnas.0711453105

[46] Choi J, Hyun Y, Kang MJ, In Yun H, Yun JY, Lister C, Dean C, Amasino RM, Noh B, Noh YS, Choi Y. Resetting and regulation of *Flowering Locus C* expression during Arabidopsis reproductive development. The Plant Journal. 2009;**57**:918-931. DOI: 10.1111/j.1365-313X.2008.03776.x

[47] Crevillén P, Yang H, Cui X, Greeff C, Trick M, Qiu Q, Cao X, Dean C. Epigenetic reprogramming that prevents transgenerational inheritance of the vernalized state. Nature. 2014;**515**:587-590. DOI: 10.1038/nature13722

[48] Tao Z, Shen L, Gu X, Wang Y, Yu H, He Y. Embryonic epigenetic reprogramming by a pioneer transcription factor in plants. Nature. 2017;**551**:124-128. DOI: 10.1038/nature24300

[49] Swiezewski S, Liu F, Magusin A, Dean C. Cold-induced silencing by long antisense transcripts of an *Arabidopsis* Polycomb target. Nature. 2009;**462**:799-802. DOI: 10.1038/nature08618

[50] Helliwell CA, Robertson M, Finnegan EJ, Buzas DM, Dennis ES. Vernalization-repression of Arabidopsis *FLC* requires promoter sequences but not antisense transcripts. PLoS One. 2011;**6**:e21513. DOI: 10.1371/journal.pone.0021513

[51] Angel A, Song J, Dean C, Howard M. A polycomb-based switch underlying quantitative epigenetic memory. Nature. 2011;**476**:105-108. DOI: 10.1038/nature10241

[52] Liu F, Marquardt S, Lister C, Swiezewski S, Dean C. Targeted 3′ processing of antisense transcripts triggers *Arabidopsis FLC* chromatin silencing. Science. 2010;**327**:94-97. DOI: 10.1126/science.1180278

[53] Sun Q, Csorba T, Skourti-Stathaki K, Proudfoot NJ, Dean C. R-loop stabilization represses antisense transcription at the *Arabidopsis FLC* locus. Science. 2013;**340**:619-621. DOI: 10.1126/science. 1234848

[54] Heo JB, Sung S. Vernalization-mediated epigenetic silencing by a long intronic noncoding RNA. Science. 2011;**331**:76-79. DOI: 10.1126/science.1197349

[55] Kim DH, Xi Y, Sung S. Modular function of long noncoding RNA, COLDAIR, in the vernalization response. PLoS Genetics. 2017;**13**:e1006939. DOI: 10.1371/journal.pgen.1006939

[56] Kim DH, Sung S. Vernalization-triggered intragenic chromatin loop formation by long noncoding RNAs. Developmental Cell. 2017;**40**:302-312. DOI: 10.1016/j.devcel.2016.12.021

[57] Zou X, Suppanz I, Raman H, Hou J, Wang J, Long Y, Jung C, Meng J. Comparative analysis of *FLC* homologues in Brassicaceae provides insight into their role in the evolution of oilseed rape. PLoS One. 2012;**7**:e45751. DOI: 10.1371/journal.pone.0045751

[58] Shea DJ, Itabashi E, Takada S, Fukai E, Kakizaki T, Fujimoto R, Okazaki K. The role of *FLOWERING LOCUS C* in vernalisation of *Brassica*: the importance of vernalisation research in the face of climate change. Crop & Pasture Science. 2018;**69**:30-39. DOI: 10.1071/CP16468

[59] Teutonico RA, Osborn TC. Mapping of RFLP and quantitative trait loci in *Brassica rapa* and comparison to linkage maps of *B. napus, B. oleracea* and *Arabidopsis*. Theoretical and Applied Genetics. 1996;**89**:885-894. DOI: 10.1007/BF00224514

[60] Osborn TC, Kole C, Parkin IAP, Sharpe AG, Kuiper M, Lydiate DJ, Trick M. Comparison of flowering time genes in *Brassica rapa, B. napus* and *Arabidopsis thaliana*. Genetics. 1997;**146**:1123-1129

[61] Kole C, Quijada P, Michaels SD, Amasino RM, Osborn TC. Evidence for homology of flowering-time genes *VFR2* from *Brassica rapa* and *FLC* from *Arabidopsis thaliana*. Theoretical and Applied Genetics. 2001;**102**:425-430. DOI: 10.1007/s001220051663

[62] Schranz ME, Quijada P, Sung SB, Lukens L, Amasino R, Osborn TC. Characterization and effects of the replicated flowering time gene *FLC* in *Brassica rapa*. Genetics. 2002;**162**:1457-1468

[63] Lou P, Zhao J, Kim JS, Shen S, Del Carpio DP, Song X, Jin M, Vreugdenhil D, Wang X, Koornneef M, Bonnema G. Quantitative trait loci for flowering time and morphological traits in multiple populations of *Brassica rapa*. Journal of Experimental Botany. 2007;**58**:4005-4016. DOI: 10.1093/jxb/erm255

[64] Li F, Kitashiba H, Inaba K, Nishio T. A *Brassica rapa* linkage map of EST-based SNP markers for identification of candidate genes controlling flowering time and leaf morphological traits. DNA Research. 2009;**16**:311-323. DOI: 10.1093/dnares/dsp020

[65] Zhao J, Kulkarni V, Liu N, Del Carpio DP, Bucher J, Bonnema G. *BrFLC2* (*FLOWERING LOCUS C*) as a candidate gene for a vernalization response QTL in *Brassica rapa*. Journal of Experimental Botany. 2010;**61**:1817-1825. DOI: 10.1093/jxb/erq048

[66] Xiao D, Zhao JJ, Hou XL, Basnet RK, Carpio DP, Zhang NW, Bucher J, Lin K, Cheng F, Wang XW, Bonnema G. The *Brassica rapa FLC* homologue *FLC2* is a key regulator of flowering time, identified through transcriptional co-expression networks. Journal of Experimental Botany. 2013;**64**:4503-4516. DOI: 10.1093/jxb/ert264

[67] Zhang X, Meng L, Liu B, Hu Y, Cheng F, Liang J, MGM A, Wang X, Wu J. A transposon insertion in *FLOWERING LOCUS T* is associated with delayed flowering in *Brassica rapa*. Plant Science. 2016;**241**:211-220. DOI: 10.1016/j.plantsci.2015.10.007

[68] Kakizaki T, Kato T, Fukino N, Ishida M, Hatakeyama K, Matsumoto S. Identification of quantitative trait loci controlling late bolting in Chinese cabbage (*Brassica rapa* L.) parental line Nou 6 gou. Breeding Science. 2011;**61**:151-159. DOI: 10.1270/jsbbs.61.151

[69] Kitamoto N, Yui S, Nishikawa K, Takahata Y, Yokoi S. A naturally occurring long insertion in the first intron in the *Brassica rapa FLC2* gene causes delayed bolting. Euphytica. 2014;**196**:213-223. DOI: 10.1007/s10681-013-1025-9

[70] Kitamoto N, Nishikawa K, Tanimura Y, Urushibara S, Matsuura T, Yokoi S, Takahata Y, Yui S. Development of late-bolting F_1 hybrids of Chinese cabbage (*Brassica rapa* L.) allowing early spring cultivation without heating. Euphytica. 2017;**213**:292. DOI: 10.1007/s10681-017-2079-x

[71] Okazaki K, Sakamoto K, Kikuchi R, Saito A, Togashi E, Kuginuki Y, Matsumoto S, Hirai M. Mapping and characterization of *FLC* homologs and QTL analysis of flowering time in *Brassica oleracea*. Theoretical and Applied Genetics. 2007;**114**:595-608. DOI: 10.1007/s00122-006-0460-6

[72] Razi H, Howell EC, Newbury HJ, Kearsey MJ. Does sequence polymorphism of *FLC* paralogues underlie flowering time QTL in *Brassica oleracea*? Theoretical and Applied Genetics. 2008;**116**:179-192. DOI: 10.1007/s00122-007-0657-3

[73] Irwin JA, Soumpourou E, Lister C, Ligthart JD, Kennedy S, Dean C. Nucleotide polymorphism affecting *FLC* expression underpins heading date variation in horticultural brassicas. The Plant Journal. 2016;**87**:597-605. DOI: 10.1111/tpj.13221

[74] Ferreira ME, Satagopan J, Yandell BS, Williams PH, Osborn TC. Mapping loci controlling vernalization requirement and flowering time in *Brassica napus*. Theoretical and Applied Genetics. 1995;**90**:727-732. DOI: 10.1007/BF00222140

[75] Wang J, Long Y, Wu B, Liu J, Jiang C, Shi L, Zhao J, King GJ, Meng J. The evolution of *Brassica napus FLOWERING LOCUS T* paralogues in the context of inverted chromosomal duplication blocks. BMC Evolutionary Biology. 2009;**9**:271. DOI: 10.1186/1471-2148-9-271

[76] Wang N, Qian W, Suppanz I, Wei L, Mao B, Long Y, Meng J, Müller AE, Jung C. Flowering time variation in oilseed rape (*Brassica napus L.*) is associated with allelic variation in the *FRIGIDA* homologue *BnaA.FRI. a*. Journal of Experimental Botany. 2011;**62**:5641-5658. DOI: 10.1093/jxb/err249

[77] Raman H, Raman R, Eckermann P, Coombes N, Manoli S, Zou X, Edwards D, Meng J, Prangnell R, Stiller J, Batley J, Luckett D, Wratten N, Dennis E. Genetic and physical mapping of flowering time loci in canola (*Brassica napus* L.). PLoS One. 2013;**126**:119-132. DOI: 10.1007/s00122-012-1966-8

[78] Raman H, Dalton-Morgan J, Diffey S, Raman R, Alamery S, Edwards D, Batley J. SNP markers-based map construction and genome-wide linkage analysis in *Brassica napus*. Plant Biotechnology Journal. 2014;**12**:851-860. DOI: 10.1111/pbi.12186

[79] Schiessl S, Iniguez-Luy F, Qian W, Snowdon RJ. Diverse regulatory factors associate with flowering time and yield responses in winter-type *Brassica napus*. BMC Genomics. 2015;**16**:737. DOI: 10.1186/s12864-015-1950-1

[80] Irwin JA, Lister C, Soumpourou E, Zhang Y, Howell EC, Teakle G, Dean C. Functional alleles of the flowering time regulator *FRIGIDA* in the *Brassica oleracea* genome. BMC Plant Biology. 2012;**12**:21. DOI: 10.1186/1471-2229-12-21

[81] Yuan YX, Wu J, Sun RF, Zhang XW, Xu DH, Bonnema G, Wang XW. A naturally occurring splicing site mutation in the *Brassica rapa FLC1* gene is associated with variation in flowering time. Journal of Experimental Botany. 2009;**60**:1299-1308. DOI: 10.1093/jxb/erp010

[82] Ridge S, Brown PH, Hecht V, Driessen RG, Weller JL. The role of *BoFLC2* in cauliflower (*Brassica oleracea* var. *botrytis* L.) reproductive development. Journal of Experimental Botany. 2015;**66**:125-135. DOI: 10.1093/jxb/eru408

[83] Tadege M, Sheldon CC, Helliwell CA, Stoutjesdijk P, Dennis ES, Peacock WJ. Control of flowering time by *FLC* orthologues in *Brassica napus*. The Plant Journal. 2011;**28**:545-553. DOI: 10.1046/j.1365-313X.2001.01182. x

[84] Kim SY, Park BS, Kwon SJ, Kim J, Lim MH, Park YD, Kim DY, Suh SC, Jin YM, Ahn JH, Lee YH. Delayed flowering time in *Arabidopsis* and *Brassica rapa* by the overexpression of *FLOWERING LOCUS C* (*FLC*) homologs isolated from Chinese cabbage (*Brassica rapa* L. ssp. *pekinensis*). Plant Cell Reports. 2007;**26**:327-336. DOI: 10.1007/s00299-006-0243-1

[85] Kawanabe T, Osabe K, Itabashi E, Okazaki K, Dennis ES, Fujimoto R. Development of primer sets that can verify the enrichment of histone modifications, and their application to examining vernalization-mediated chromatin changes in *Brassica rapa* L. Genes & Genetic Systems. 2016;**91**:1-10. DOI: 10.1266/ggs.15-00058

[86] Sheldon CC, Conn AB, Dennis ES, Peacock WJ. Different regulatory regions are required for the vernalization-induced repression of *FLOWERING LOCUS C* and for the epigenetic maintenance of repression. The Plant Cell. 2002;**14**:2527-2537. DOI: 10.1105/tpc.004564

[87] Tsai MC, Manor O, Wan Y, Mosammaparast N, Wang JK, Lan F, Shi Y, Segal E, Chang HY. Long noncoding RNA as modular scaffold of histone modification complexes. Science. 2010;**329**:689-693. DOI: 10.1126/science.1192002.Long

[88] Li X, Zhang S, Bai J, He Y. Tuning growth cycles of *Brassica* crops via natural antisense transcripts of *BrFLC*. Plant Biotechnology Journal. 2016;**14**:905-914. DOI: 10.1111/pbi.12443

Chapter 7

Benefits of Entomophile Pollination in Crops of *Brassica napus* and Aspects of Plant Floral Biology

Emerson D. Chambó, Simone C. Camargo,
Regina C. Garcia, Carlos A.L. Carvalho,
Maria Claudia C. Ruvolo-Takasusuki,
Ludimilla Ronqui, Claudio Silva Júnior,
Pedro R. Santos and
Vagner de Alencar Arnaut de Toledo

Additional information is available at the end of the chapter

http://dx.doi.org/10.5772/intechopen.74569

Abstract

Rapeseed (*Brassica napus* L. var. oleifera) is an oleaginous species of the Brassicaceae family, being the third most produced oleaginous in the world. Rapeseed can produce fruits and seeds from both self-pollination and cross-pollination. However, cross-pollination rate is approximately 30% and may suffer variations due to the abundance and diversity of pollinator insects, cultivar and meteorological conditions. Different researchers have reported that pollination by insects, especially *Apis mellifera* honeybee, on rapeseed flowers provides an increase in productivity, improving yield and contributing to the uniformity and initial pod establishment. It is estimated that the economic value of *A. mellifera* honeybees for rapeseed cultivation in Brazil is US$ 8.2 million. The objective of this chapter is gathering data for a compilation of information regarding rapeseed culture and the importance of *A. mellifera* in *Brassica napus* pollination.

Keywords: canola, oil, pod, pollination, seed

1. Introduction

1.1. History and botanical origin

Rapeseed is a plant of the Brassicaceae family, belonging to the *Brassica* genus. This plant was developed by conventional genetic breeding of rapeseed, which allowed the reduction of erucic acid levels and glucosinolates that are toxic to humans. That is why the word canola, a derivation of an English term "CANadian Oil Low Acid" that refers to the generic cultivars of rape that meet the specific standards regarding the levels of these substances. Rapeseed was registered in Canada in 1970, and today its name is used to designate three species of *Brassica*: *B. napus* or Argentine variety, *B. rapa*, also known as Polish and *B. juncea* or mustard [1].

Taxonomic studies carried out in the 1930s showed that *B. carinata*, *B. juncea* and *B. napus* are alotetraploid species formed by hybridization events between diploid parent species *B. nigra*, *B. rapa* and *B. oleracea*. Hybridization between *B. nigra* and *B. oleracea* resulted in the formation of *B. carinata*; between *B. nigra* and *B. rapa* in *B. juncea* formation and between *B. oleracea* and *B. rapa* in *B. napus* [2].

Haploid genomes of *B. rapa*, *B. nigra* and *B. oleracea* are designated A, B and C, respectively. Thus, *B. rapa* diploids have two copies of the genome A on 20 chromosomes (AA, n = 10, 2n = 20), and *B. napus* diploids have two copies of both genomes A and C on 38 chromosomes (AACC, n = 19, 2n = 38), see **Figure 1**.

Mitochondrial DNA and chloroplasts analysis suggested that *B. montana* (n = 9) might be closely related to the prototype that gave rise to both *B. rapa* and *B. oleracea* cytoplasms. Furthermore, results from phylogenetic analyses have shown that there are multiple origins of *B. napus* and that the most cultivated forms of this species derived from a crossing where a closely related ancestral species of *B. rapa* and *B. oleracea* was the maternal donor [3].

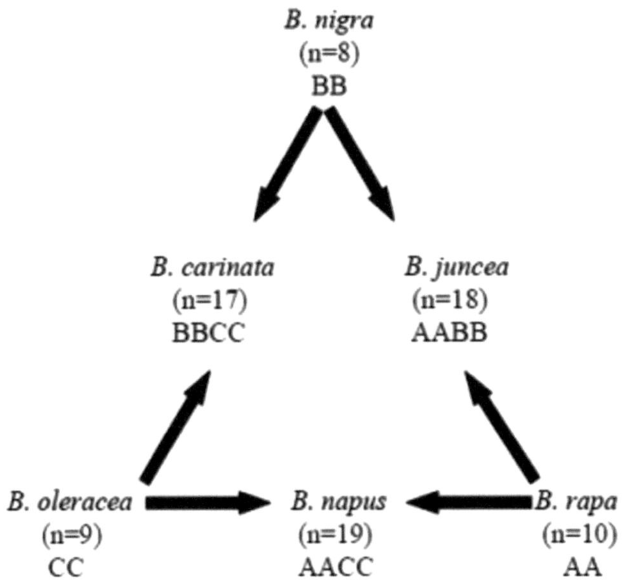

Figure 1. Nagaharu [2] triangle illustrating the genomic relations between Brassica species. The haploid genomes of the diploid species of *B. rapa*, *B. nigra* and *B. oleracea* are referred to as A, B and C, respectively.

2. Floral biology aspects

B. napus flowers are bisexual, have four sepals, four petals, four long stamens and two short stamens on the same flower. The anthers present longitudinal dehiscence. The ovary is superimposed, with parietal placentation, gamocarpelar and bicarpelar. There are nectaries located in the center of the flower, two between the ovary and the two short stamens, and two between the two long stamens and the petals [4].

Anthesis in rapeseed flowers can occur at any time of the day, but usually occurs early in the morning, around 9 am, when most of them are already open. The flowers remain open for up to 3 days, and at night they partially close and the opening occurs again the following morning. Winter rapeseed flowers remain open for one to 3 days, while spring rapeseed flowers remain open for 1–2 days. Flowering, which lasts from 22 to 45 days, depends on the weather conditions [5, 6]. For example, when the weather is cold and humid, flowers stay open longer for hotter and drier days [7].

In cultivars of the auto sterile *Brassica* genus, anthers of the long stamens release the pollen into the environment, and cross-pollination is essential. On the other hand, in some auto sterile cultivars, the release of the pollen begins even before the opening of the flower and continues until the end of the anthesis. In these cultivars, during the flowering period the stigma reaches the position of the long stamens, while the anthers initially release the pollen into the environment and then curl up for some pollen to be directed to the stigma of the same flower. In other cultivars, mainly those that produce yellow seeds, the pollen grains produced in the anthers are deposited on the stigma of the same flower, leading to self-pollination [5].

The stigmatic surface is receptive to the pollen for up to 3 days after anthesis. If the temperature is high, above 27°C, almost all pollen grains are released on the first day of anthesis, the time the flower becomes receptive to the pollen and the viability of the pollen is decreased. The most favorable temperature for rapeseed cultivation is around 20°C during the cycle. Fertilization occurs within 24 hours after pollination, and fertilization, the flower remains partially closed and the petals begin to peel (2 to 3 days after flower opening). The young pod becomes visible in the center of the flower 1 day after the fall of the petals [8].

Another important factor in rapeseed concerns the fertilization of the ovules, especially the percentage of ovules with complete embryo sacs in the opening of the flower. Even with a large deposition of pollen on the stigma, incomplete pollination may occur. In rapeseed, generally 30% of the eggs are sterile due to the absence of complete embryo sacs in the opening of the flower. The lower proportion of ovules with complete embryo bags will result in a non-fertilization of all the ovules of the flower and, consequently, a smaller number of seeds per pod [9]. In the terminal raceme, the lower proportion of fertile ovules due to the sterility of the ovules and the lower number of ovules per ovary in apical flowers are some of the causes for the smaller number of seeds per pod in the apical region compared to the basal region [10].

The life cycle of the rapeseed plant is divided into seven main stages: germination (stage 0), foliar development (stage 1), development of lateral branches (stage 2), stem elongation (stage 3), inflorescence emergence (stage 4), flowering (stage 5), seed development (stage 6) and maturation (stage 7). Knowledge of the stages of development of the rapeseed plant is important for decision-making and crop management. However, the beginning of each stage of development is not dependent on the end of the previous step. From the beginning of flowering, each stage of growth is determined by analyzing the main flowering stem. The timing and occurrence of the different stages of growth will vary according to the conditions of growth, location and variety used in the crop [8].

3. Pollination requirements in rapeseed flowers

In many plant species, pollination is essential for sexual reproduction. Many floral characteristics are adaptations to promote cross-pollination and have evolved to reduce the negative impact of inbreeding depression and increase the likelihood of male success [11].

The flowers pollinated by animals usually have attractive petals and offer floral reward such as nectar or pollen [5, 12]. However, visits by pollinators may sometimes not involve plant needs and seed production may be limited by the amount of pollen deposited on the stigma [13].

In plants with hermaphrodite and self-compatible flowers, such as *B. napus*, self-pollination can offer reproductive guarantee when there is a shortage of visits of pollinating agents. Mixed mating systems, which include self-pollination, are therefore adaptive [14], although there may be detrimental consequences due to inbreeding depression [15].

However, in rapeseed, pollinator insects, especially *Apis mellifera* honeybees, may play an important role in pollination and are believed to be involved in pollen transfer over long distances [16]. Honeybees combined with other bee species may result in better pollination than any single insect population [17].

Rapeseed has flowers capable of both self-pollination and cross-pollination, although under field conditions the fertilization of the ovules of their flowers usually results, for the most part, from self-pollination [1, 16]. The cross-pollination rate, which in canola is approximately 30%, may suffer variations due to the abundance and diversity of pollinator insects, cultivar and meteorological conditions [1, 18].

Despite higher self-pollination rate compared to cross-pollination in rapeseed, higher seed production has been reported when pollinated by bees [19–23]. Rapeseed flowers secrete large amounts of nectar and are very attractive to *A. mellifera* honeybees and other pollinating insects [5, 6].

In addition, in rapeseed, in spite of the autogamy, mechanisms for occurrence of allogamy were found from reproductive strategies used by this species, such as abundant pollen, nectar and odor. These mechanisms were important for the genetic breeding of the species, favoring the occurrence of more adaptive characteristics [4].

Although data are still conflicting and divergent among rapeseed varieties on the benefits of entomophile pollination, there is evidence that insects can qualitatively and quantitatively increase crop production. The interdependence of bees and the *Brassica* genus are manifested in the fact that their pollen is very sticky and there is a need for pollen insects for their transfer. For *Brassica spp.* plants, bees are co-evolved in pollen transfer mechanisms [24].

Self-pollinating can promote seed production, but for this, viable pollen must contact stigma when it is receptive. The degree of self-polishing would be greatest when the stigma is pushed up through the anthers. However, if time, pollen availability or stigma receptivity is not synchronized, seed production will not occur [25].

Entomophile pollination efficiency process depends mainly on the climatic conditions, as it also affects the crop as well as the pollinators [24]. High temperatures in the pre-anthesis may cause pollen sterility, and in the anthesis, delayed growth of the pollen tube [26], as well as high temperatures and low relative humidity may lead to a decrease in stigma receptivity [27] and degeneration of flower ovules [28]. Thus, understanding the role of pollinators and factors affecting insect–plant interactions may be of great importance for increasing grain yield in rapeseed.

In addition, it should be considered that most *Brassica* species are self-incompatible; therefore, insect visits are necessary for seed production [6, 29]. In *Brassica* species with auto incompatibility (AI), incompatible pollen grains barely germinate on stigma and, when germinated, their pollen tubes fail to grow on papillary cells on the stigmatic surface [30]. Self-incompatibility is a widespread mechanism in flowering plants that prevent self-fertilization. Self-pollen recognition is located at the *S* locus. Pollen rejection occurs when the same *S* allele is expressed both by the pollen and the pistil tissues. This suggests that the *S*-locus encoding the male determinant and another encoding the female component of the Self-incompatibility reaction [31].

In rapeseed, the stigma can accumulate pollen in the absence of pollinating insects from the pollen of its own anthers by spontaneous self-pollination by mechanical contact caused by flower collisions or anemophilic pollination, as well as by cross-pollination [32]. In lower pollinator densities, rapeseed seed production occurs through the spontaneous auto-pollination mechanism in the flower and the mechanical contact caused by collisions between flowers or anemophilous pollination.

On the other hand, in moderate bees densities, non-insect pollination modes and entomophile pollination also contribute to seed production. Even at the highest levels of pollinator abundance found in crop fields, spontaneous self-pollination accounts for almost a third of production [32]. In this context, the dynamics of pollen transfer mediated by bees must be considered to be dependent on the amount of pollen available, as well as on pollen removal rates from anther and deposition on the stigma by specific pollinators [33].

Pollinators with high removal and low pollen deposition (HRLD) on flower stigmas will benefit a plant species when there is no better pollinator available. Pollinators with high pollen removal and high deposition (HRHD) on stigmas may have a decrease in total pollen transfer as a result of visits by HRLD pollinators. HRLDs parasitize plants by diverting the grains that would be delivered by HRHDs. In situations where two visitors remove equal amounts of pollen, the one with the highest deposition rate will always be a more efficient pollinator; if it removes different amounts, which is better not only depend on deposition rates, but on other variables such as visitation frequency for deposition [33].

4. Impact of pollination by honeybees on *B. napus*

Commercially grown rapeseed hybrids are predominantly auto-fertile, but the degree of cross-pollination is still uncertain [34]. In cultures that are poorly dependent on pollinators, such as rapeseed, introduction of honeybee colonies is generally not recommended [35]. However, as long as the flowers of these hybrids are attractive to the pollinators, the introduction of 3–5 colonies of *A. mellifera* or 5–8 colonies of *A. cerana* uniformly distributed per hectare may be ideal for increasing production and higher oil content of the seeds [33]. There is evidence that pollination by honeybees in rapeseed provides increased productivity, improving yield and contributing to the uniformity and initial pod establishment [24, 36].

In *B. napus* the number of pods per plant may decrease by 16% in plants located at a distance of 1.000 m from the apiary [20]. Manning and Wallis [37] found grain yield 20% or 400 kg.ha^{-1} higher in plots located close to the apiary than those located at a distance of 200 m from the apiary. Pordel et al. [38] reported that pollinating insects, especially *A. mellifera,* more abundant in rapeseed crops, could increase grain yield by 53%.

The influence of honeybee density on rapeseed production in nine agricultural fields with three honeybee densities: 0, 1.5 and 3.0 colonies/hectare was evaluated. The results of this experiment indicated an increase in the seed productivity of 46% in the presence of three colonies per hectare in relation to the absent area of pollinators [21].

Araneda-Durán et al. [22] evaluated *B. napus* cv. Artus production pollinated by *A. mellifera* from an experiment that consisted of three treatments: exclusion of pollinators from rapeseed plants, partial exclusion and free pollination with a density of 6.5 colonies/hectare. The results evidenced increase of seed productivity induced by the treatment with free pollination of 50.34% on the total exclusion and 11.46% in relation to the partial exclusion.

One the one hand, in the Hyola 433 and 61 rapeseed cultivars it was observed that insect pollination was higher for the variables number of pods per plant, number of seeds per pod and average pod weight, respectively, in the condition of autogamy [23]. In CTC-4 rapeseed cultivar, visits of honeybees collecting nectar and pollen contributed to increase pod production per square meter and mass of each grain. However, no influence was recorded on the total number of seeds per pod normal and abnormal seeds per pod, germination and oil content in seeds [39].

Therefore, divergent results were obtained in an experiment carried out with the CTC-4 rapeseed cultivar in Dourados, Brazil. In this experiment, there were no statistically significant differences when the free-pollination and autogamy treatments were compared for the variables pod size, number of seeds per pod and weight of 10 pods [4].

It should be considered that the productivity of rapeseed seeds is a function of population density, number of pods per plant, number of seeds per pod and seed weight. Besides, the numbers of pods per plant being the most important variable for increase in grain yield, especially in crops with low plant densities and non-uniform populations [40].

5. Situation and economic aspects

Rapeseed is a kind of cold climate; therefore, its commercial cultivation in the world is concentrated in temperate regions, mainly in latitudes higher than 35°C [41]. Air temperature and water availability are the most important environmental variables for its growth and development [42].

Most of the rapeseed produced in Europe is of the winter type, however, in Brazil there are only spring rapeseed and from *Brassica napus* L. species. This is because even in the coldest conditions in Brazil, as in State of Rio Grande do Sul, the number of hours required for winter cultivars is insufficient [43].

Its cultivation is mainly due to its seeds, which produce between 35% and 45% of oil. The main use of rapeseed is like cooking oil, but it is also commonly used in margarine. Rapeseed meal is produced as a by-product during the oil extraction from the seeds and used as a source of high protein content intended for animal feed [1]. In addition, rapeseed is an excellent alternative for crop rotation with grasses and vegetables, as well as being appropriately inserted in the cultivation systems that predominate in the South of Brazil [44].

Currently, rapeseed accounts for 15% of vegetable oil production, behind soybeans (28.6%) and palm (33.2%), as well as being the third largest commodity in the world [45]. The main world producers in the 2011/2012 harvests were the European Union, Canada, China and India. World production of rapeseed seed in the 2011/2012 harvests was projected at 60.93 million tons, at 33.76 million hectares of planted area [46].

In Brazil, rapeseed grains production in the 2011/2012 harvests was 52 thousand tons, in 42.400 hectares of planted area; with State of Rio Grande do Sul being the largest producer, followed by the State of Paraná [47]. Producers have harvested, on average, 20.44 sacks per hectare or the equivalent of 1226.00 $kg.ha^{-1}$, with production costs of R$ 1310.00 per hectare. The price of the 60 kg bag of rapeseed marketed in August 2012 was R$ 72.66 [48]. Therefore, the gross revenue of the crop can be estimated at approximately R$ 62.9 million, with net sales of R$ 7.4 million.

Bees are the most important and economically most valuable pollinators in the world. Many crops of economic interest, such as oilseeds, are dependent, at least in part, on pollination by these insects. The evidence for this is that in 2005, the world economic value of pollination services totaled € 153 billion, representing 9.5% of the economic value of world agricultural production used for human consumption [49]. In the United States alone, in 2000, the benefit of honeybee pollination services totaled US$ 14.6 billion [50].

The economic value of *A. mellifera* honeybees for rapeseed cultivation in Brazil can be simulated in order to determine the contribution of the Africanized honeybees to the total economic value of the oilseed production. This estimation can be performed from the $Vhb = V \times D \times P$ Eq. [50, 51], where Vhb is the annual value of the crop attributed to *A. mellifera* honeybees; V is the value of the rapeseed production in grains in the 2011/2012 crop, published by [48]; D is the culture dependence by pollinator animals of 0.25 [49]; P is the effective proportion of pollinating insects that are *A. mellifera* L., obtained by [50] of 0.90. Therefore, Vhb = 62.9 × 0.25 × 0.90 = R$ 14.2 million or about US $ 8 million.

Thus, the amount of R$ 14.2 million attributed to honeybees represents that the pollination services of rapeseed deserve further investigation due to the lack of knowledge about the pollination requirements of the various hybrids commercialized in Brazil. In addition, the benefit generated by honeybees may change due to climatic conditions and the hybrid used, which indicates once again the importance of understanding the possible factors that may affect the pollination process performed by these insects.

In addition, the growing demand from the productive sectors increases the area cultivated with rapeseed in Brazil, despite the slight drop in production caused by unsatisfactory environmental conditions. Currently, most of the Brazilian crops occur in States of Rio Grande do Sul and Paraná, with some crops in States of Mato Grosso do Sul and Santa Catarina. Brazilian producers are improving technical knowledge on cultivation and harvesting, improving the final results of the harvest [45].

Acknowledgements

To CNPq (National Council for Scientific and Technological Development), process number 311663/2014-1 for the financial support, and CAPES (Coordination of Improvement of Higher Level Personnel) for the scholarship for the first author.

Author details

Emerson D. Chambó[1], Simone C. Camargo[2], Regina C. Garcia[3], Carlos A.L. Carvalho[4], Maria Claudia C. Ruvolo-Takasusuki[5], Ludimilla Ronqui[6], Claudio Silva Júnior[2], Pedro R. Santos[2] and Vagner de Alencar Arnaut de Toledo[2]*

*Address all correspondence to: vagner_abelha@yahoo.co.uk

1 Nature and Culture Institute, Federal University of Amazonas, Benjamin Constant, Brazil

2 Animal Science Department, Maringá State University, Maringá, Brazil

3 Agrarian Sciences Center, Western of Paraná State University, Marechal Cândido Rondon, Brazil

4 Insecta Research Group, Agrarian Sciences, Environmental, and Biological Center, Federal University of Recôncavo of Bahia, Cruz das Almas, Brazil

5 Cellular Biology, Genetics, and Biotechnology Department, Maringá State University, Maringá, Brazil

6 Federal University of Paraná, Palotina, Brazil

References

[1] Office of the Gene Technology Regulator (OGTR). Biology of *Brassica napus* L. (Canola). Australian: OGTR; 2011

[2] Nagaharu U. Genome analysis in *Brassica* with special reference to the experimental formation of *B. napus* and peculiar mode of fertilization. Journal of Japanese Botany. 1935;**7**:389-452

[3] Song K, Osborn TC. Polyphyletic origins of *Brassica napus*: New evidence based on organelle and nuclear RFLP analyses. Genome. 1992;**35**:992-1001. DOI: 10.1139/g92-152

[4] Mussury RM, Fernandes WD. Studies of the floral biology and reproductive system of *Brassica napus* L. (Cruciferae). Brazilian Archives of Biology and Technology. 2000;**43**:111-115. DOI: 10.1590/S1516-89132000000100014

[5] Free JB. Insect Pollination of Crops, 2nd ed. London, UK: Academic Press; 1993. 849 p

[6] Delaplane KS, Mayer DF. Crop Pollination by Bees. New York, NY: CABI Publishing; 2000. 352 p

[7] Williams I. The pollination of Swede rape (*Brassica napus* L.). Bee World. 1985;**66**:16-22

[8] Thomas P. Canola Grower's Manual. Winnipeg, Canada: Canola Council of Canada; 2003

[9] Wang X, Mathieu A, Cournède PH, Allirand JM, Jullien A, Reffye P, Zhang BG. Stochastic models in floral biology and its application to the study of oilseed rape (*Brassica napus* L.) fertility. In: Li B, Guo Y, Jaeger M, editors. Proceedings, Symposium: The Third International Symposium on Plant Growth Modeling, Simulation, Visualization and Applications (PMA 09), Nov 9-13, 2009. Beijing, China: INRIA; 2010. pp. 175-182. DOI: 10.1109/PMA.2009.12

[10] Bouttier C, Morgan DG. Ovule development and determination of seed number per pod in oilseed rape (*Brassica napus* L.). Journal of Experimental Botany. 1992;**42**:109-714. DOI: 10.1093/jxb/43.5.709

[11] Barrett SCH. The evolution of plant sexual diversity. Nature Reviews Genetics. 2002;**3**:274-284

[12] McGregor SE. Insect Pollination of Cultivated Crop Plants. USDA, Washington, DC; 1976. 849 p

[13] Wilcock C, Neiland R. Pollination failure in plants: Why it happens and when it matters. Trends in Plant Science. 2002;**7**:270-277. DOI: 10.1016/S1360-1385(02)02258-6

[14] Morgan MT, Wilson WG. Self-fertilization and the escape from pollen limitation in variable pollination environments. Evolution. 2005;**59**:1143-1148

[15] Cresswell JE. The influence of nectar and pollen availability on pollen transfer by individual flowers of oil-seed rape (*Brassica napus*) when pollinated by bumblebees (*Bombus lapidarius*). Journal of Ecology. 1999;**87**:670-677. DOI: 10.1046/j.1365-2745.1999.00385.x

[16] Environmental Health and Safety Publications (OCDE). Consensus Document on the Biology of *Brassica napus* L. (Oilseed Rape). France: OECD; 1997

[17] DeGrandi-Hoffman G, Watkins JC. The foraging activity of honey bees *Apis mellifera* and non-*Apis* bees on hybrid sunflower (*Helianthus annuus*) and its influence on cross-pollination and seed set. Journal of Apicultural Research. 2000;**39**:37-45. DOI: 10.1080/00218839.2000.11101019

[18] Canadian Food Inspection Agency (CFIA). The Biology of *Brassica napus*. Canadá: Plant Biosafety Office; 1999

[19] Williams IH, Martin AP, White RP. The effect of insect pollination on plant development and seed production in winter oil-seed rape (*Brassica napus* L.). Journal of Agricultural Science. 1987;**109**:135-139. DOI: 10.1017/S0021859600081077

[20] Manning R, Boland J. A preliminary investigation into honey bee (*Apis mellifera*) pollination of canola (*Brassica napus* cv Karoo). Australian Journal of Experimental Agriculture. 2000;**40**:439-442. DOI: 10.1071/EA98148

[21] Sabbahi R, Oliveira D, Marceau J. Influence of honey bee (Hymenoptera: Apidae) density on the production of canola (Cruciferae: Brassicaceae). Journal of Economic Entomology. 2005;**98**:367-372

[22] Araneda-Durán X, Ulloa RB, Carrillo JA, Contreras JL, Bastidas MT. Evaluation of yield component traits of honeybee-pollinated (*Apis mellifera* L.) rapeseed canola (*Brassica napus* L.). Chilean Journal of Agricultural Research. 2010;**70**:309-314. DOI: 10.1051/apido:19920302

[23] Chambó ED, Oliveira NTE, Garcia RC, Duarte-Júnior JB, Ruvolo-Takasusuki MCC, Arnaut de Toledo VA. Pollination of rapeseed (*Brassica napus*) by Africanized honeybees (Hymenoptera: Apidae) on two sowing dates. Anais da Academia Brasileira de Ciências. 2014;**86**(4):2087-2100. DOI: 10.1590/0001-3765201420140134

[24] Abrol DP. Honeybees and rapeseed: A pollinator-plant interaction. Advances in Botanical Research. 2007;**45**:337-367. DOI: 10.1016/S0065-2296(07)45012-1

[25] DeGrandi-Hoffman G, Chambers M. Effects of honey bee (Hymenoptera: Apidae) foraging on seed set in self-fertile sunflowers (*Helianthus annuus* L.). Environmental Entomology. 2006;**35**:1103-1108. DOI: 10.1603/0046-225X-35.4.1103

[26] Prasad PVV, Crauford PQ, Kakani VG, Wheeler TR, Boote K. Influence of high temperature during pre- and post-anthesis stages of floral development on fruit-set and pollen germination in peanut. Australian Journal of Plant Physiology. 2001;**28**:233-240. DOI: 10.1071/PP0012

[27] Hedhly A, Hormaza JI, Herrero M. Effect of temperature on pollen tube kinetics and dynamics in sweet cherry, *Prunus avium* (Rosaceae). American Journal of Botany. 2004;**91**:558-564. DOI: 10.3732/ajb.91.4.558

[28] Cerovic R, Ruzic D, Micic N. Viability of plum ovules at different temperatures. Annals of Applied Biology. 2000;**137**:53-59. DOI: 10.1111/j.1744-7348.2000.tb00056.x

[29] Morandin LA, Winston ML. Wild bee abundance and seed production in conventional, organic, and genetically modified canola. Ecological Applications. 2005;**15**:871-881. DOI: 10.1890/03-5271

[30] Schifino-Wittmann MT, Dall'agnol M. Autoincompatibilidade em plantas. Ciencia Rural. 2002;**32**:1083-1090. DOI: 10.1590/S0103-84782002000600027

[31] Gaude T, Cabrillac D. Self-incompatibility in flowering plants: The *Brassica* model. Comptes rendus de l'Académie des sciences. Série III, Sciences de la vie. 2001;**324**:537-542. DOI: 10.1016/S0764-4469(01)01323-3

[32] Hoyle M, Hayter K, Cresswell JE. Effect of pollinator abundance on self-fertilization and gene flow: Application to GM canola. Ecological Applications. 2007;**17**:2123-2135

[33] Thomson JD, Goodell K. Pollen removal and deposition by honeybee and bumblebee visitors to apple and almond flowers. Journal of Applied Ecology. 2002;**38**:1032-1044. DOI: 10.1046/j.1365-2664.2001.00657.x

[34] Abrol DP. Pollination Biology: Biodiversity Conservation and Agricultural Production. New York, NY: Springer; 2012. 792 p. DOI: 10.1007/978-94-007-1942-2

[35] Cunningham S, Fitzgibbon F, Heard TA. The future of pollinators for Australian agriculture. Australian Journal of Agricultural Research. 2002;**53**:893-900. DOI: 10.1046/j.1365-2745.1999.00385.x

[36] Abrol DP, Shankar U. Pollination in oil crops: Recent advances and future strategies. In: Gupta SK, editor. Technological Innovations in Major World Oil Crops. Vol. 2. New York, NY: Springer; 2012. pp. 221-267

[37] Manning R, Wallis I. Seed yields in canola (*Brassica napus* cv. Karoo) depend on the distance of plants from honeybee apiaries. Australian Journal of Experimental Agriculture. 2005;**45**:1307-1313

[38] Pordel MR, Hatami B, Mobli M, Ebadi R. Identification of insect pollinators of three different cultivars of winter canola and their effect on seed yield in Isfahan. Journal of Science and Technology of Agricultural and Natural Resources. 2007;**10**:413-426

[39] Adegas JEB, Nogueira-Couto RH. Entomophilous pollination in rape (*Brassica napus* L. var oeifera) in Brazil. Apidologie. 1992;**23**:203-209. DOI: 10.1051/apido:19920302

[40] Angadi SV, Cutfoth HW, McConkey BG, Gan Y. Yield adjustment by canola grown at different plant populations under semiarid conditions. Crop Science. 2003;**43**:1358-1366

[41] McClinchey SL, Kott LS. Production of mutants with high cold tolerance in spring canola (*Brassica napus*). Euphytica. 2008;**162**:51-67

[42] Gan Y, Angadi SV, Cutforth H, Potts D, Angadi VV, McDonald CL. Canola and mustard response to short periods of temperature and water stress at different developmental stages. Canadian Journal of Plant Science. 2004;**84**:697-704. DOI: 10.4141/P03-109

[43] Tomm GO, Ferreira PEP, Aguiar JLP, Castro AMG, Lima SMV, Mori C. Panorama atual e indicações para o aumento de eficiência da produção de canola no Brasil. Passo Fundo, RS: Embrapa Trigo; 2009

[44] Dalmago GA, Cunha GR, Tomm GO, Pires LF, Santi A, Pasinato A, Fanton G, Luersen I, Müller FLD, Müller AL. Zoneamento agroclimático para o cultivo de canola no Rio Grande do Sul. Revista Brasileira de Agrometeorologia. 2008;**16**:295-305

[45] Companhia Nacional de Abastecimento (CONAB). Canola. Conab, Brasília, DF; 2011. Available from: http://conab.gov.br

[46] United States Department of Agriculture (USDA). World Agricultural Production. Washington, DC: USDA; 2012. Available from: http://usda01.library.cornell.edu/usda/fas/worldag-production//2010s/2011/worldag-production-05-11-2011.pdf

[47] Companhia Nacional de Abastecimento (CONAB). Acompanhamento de safra brasileira: grãos, quarto levantamento. Conab, Brasília, DF; 2013. Available from: http://conab.gov.br

[48] Companhia Nacional de Abastecimento (CONAB). Canola. Conab, Brasília, DF; 2012. Available from: http://conab.gov.br

[49] Gallai N, Salles JM, Settele J, Vaissière BE. Economic valuation of the vulnerability of world agriculture confronted with pollinator decline. Ecological Economics. 2009;**68**:810-821. DOI: 10.1016/j.ecolecon.2008.06.014

[50] Morse RA, Calderone NW. The value of honey bees as pollinators of U.S. crops in 2000. Bee Culture. 2000;**132**:1-15

[51] Robinson WS, Nowogrodzki R, Morse RA. The value of honeybees as pollinators of U.S. crops. American Bee Journal. 1989;**129**:411-423

Chapter 8

Economic Insect Pests of *Brassica*

Muhammad Imran

Additional information is available at the end of the chapter

http://dx.doi.org/10.5772/intechopen.74837

Abstract

Brassica is a genus of plants in the mustard family that includes cauliflower, sprouts, broccoli and cabbage. Plants of the *brassica* family are rich sources of biologically active substance. The beneficial effects of *brassica* vegetables on human health have been somewhat linked to phytochemicals. They prevent oxidative stress, induce detoxification enzymes, stimulate immune system and decrease the risk of cancers. Crucifers are the important winter crops grown widely in tropical and temperate regions of the world, giving yield of 50.7 million tons. It is cultivated around the year over an area of 8263 hectares in Karnataka with production of 23.63 tons per hectare. Cauliflower and cabbage are the most common crops throughout the world. Diamondback moth (DBM) caused losses of about 16 million dollars by causing a 2.5% damage annually. There are many insect pests that attacked these crops and most common are diamondback moth, tobacco cutworm, aphid, jassid, cabbage worm and many others. The most important of these insect pests is the diamondback moth *Plutella xylostella* also called cabbage moth that belongs to Plutellidae. There are many controlled strategies including chemical control, biological control, physical control and many other methods. This study contributes to the literature offering understandings about the insect pests of *brassica* and their best management techniques.

Keywords: *brassica*, insect pests, DBM, bionomic, distribution, management

1. Introduction

Cruciferous family crops are economically important, and especially cabbage (*Brassica oleracea*) is one of the most important winter vegetables grown extensively in temperate and tropical areas of the world with an output of 50.7 million tons, of which India contributes 38.62 lakh metric tons, from an area of 2.18 lakh hectares [1]. The most important of cole crops, cabbage and cauliflower, are grown on 0.438 million hectares producing 6.335 million tons per annum in India [1]. In China, cruciferous family plants are also cultivated on large areas. The most damaging pest of cruciferous family plants is diamondback moth (DBM), *Plutella xylostella* (L.) (Lepidoptera: Plutellidae) because of its greater dispersal ability, per-year larger number of generation and development of resistance to most commonly used insecticides [2, 3]. *P. xylostella* is a serious pest of cauliflower, cabbage, lily, brussels, broccoli, sprouts and Chinese cabbage [2].

2. Bionomic of diamondback moth

2.1. Biology and ecology

DBM is a tiny brownish color moth having triangular markings on their forewing. Eggs are laid signally on the underside of leaves. The female of diamondback moth lays 300 eggs in her reproductive period. The female of DBM lays eggs on the lower and upper side of the leaf surface and the ratio is 3:2, and very little amount of eggs are laid on the stems of the leaf [4]. An egg hatching period is 2–4 days. As new tiny larvae emerge, they start feeding on the lower side of leaves. Larval duration is 10–15 days but it largely depends on the temperature and other environmental conditions. Color of young larvae is from whitish yellow to pale green. The life of an adult is 10–15 days. Larvae cause large defoliation of leaves [5]. Diamondback moth adult is a weak flier and the length of adult moth is about 5 mm and width is 2 mm [6].

After the emergence, the first instar makes mines in the spongy tissue and the second instar starts feeding on the lower side of the leaf and consumes all the tissue expect the waxy layer. When fourth instar feeding is complete, it converts into a cocoon-like structure that is called the pupal stage, and at this stage feeding stops [7]. The duration of this stage depends upon the temperature and mostly it is 4–10 days, but it can decrease in warm areas and increase in cold areas; after adults emerge who feed on water or dew drops, their adult life is short [8].

2.2. Diapause

In subtropical and tropical regions, where the cabbage and cauliflower or any other crops belonging to the Crucifers family are grown throughout the year, all the stages of diamondback moth are present at any time. In the temperate region, where the crucifers crop are not grown throughout the year, and in winter season, both pupal and adult stages of diamondback moth hibernate in plant debris [9]. A study was done in the New York state for the presence of diamondback moth during winter season using different pheromone traps and it found that no diamondback moths were caught [10].

2.3. Migration

Diamondback moths have great abilities to disperse and migrate over long distances. Mass migration of DBM occurs in Britain, and the adult of diamondback moth migrates from Baltic to Southern Finland and covers about 3000 km, and this study indicates that the adult of DBM remains in flight continuously for several days [11].

3. Distribution of diamondback moth

Plutella xylostella was for the first time recorded in Europe but later found throughout America, Australia, Southeast Asia and New Zealand. For the first time, it was observed in North America in 1854, in Illinois, and then spread to Florida and the Rocky Mountains in 1883 and in 1905, diamondback moth was reported in British Columbia [2].

Diamondback moth has been recorded all over the world and the largest number of this species was recorded in the USA. Seven species of this insect was recorded in South America and Argentina, Chile and Colombia recorded nine species and only two species of *Plutella* have been recorded in Europe. The world's most important five species include *P. annulatella* (Curt.) in Finland; *P. armoraclae* (Bus.) in Colorado, the USA; *P. antiphona* (Mey.) in New Zealand; *P. porrectella* (L.) in Ontario, Canada; and *P. xylostella* (L.). All these species are limited in their geographic distribution except *P. xylostella*. It is also suggested that this pest might have originated in South Africa because the presence of rich and diverse fauna [12].

4. Damaging history of diamondback moth

Diamondback moth is a serious pest of cruciferous plants worldwide and about 1 billion dollars of losses occur annually due to its larval damage [13]. It is reported that 90% of losses occur due to this pest [14] and also reported that 60% loss occurs in production and 2 billion dollars of losses occur when controlling this pest [15]. It is estimated that 16 million dollars of losses occur on the basis of a 2.5% damage on protective crops per annum by this pest [1]. The larvae of DBM caused damage to all cruciferous family crops especially cabbage in Southeast Asia.

The failure of DBM occurred when this insect became the most destructive pest of the Lepidopteran family. DBM damaged above-ground plant parts and reduced the yield except during rainy weather [16]. When the attack of diamondback moth is very serious the losses reach up to 80–90% [17].

4.1. Mode of damage

The larvae of diamondback moth *Plutella xylostella* feed on the foliage at their different larvae stages and reduce the yield and also decrease the quality of vegetables [18]. Larvae of DBM damage the cabbage and cauliflower leaves by making small holes on the surface of leaves, often leaving the epidermis of leaves that is called Feeding Window; also, inside broccoli florets and cauliflower curds, contamination occurs due to this insect.

5. Chemical control of diamondback moth

There are many specific insecticides used for the control of DBM while certain chemicals are more effective against other pests as compared to DBM, so it is important to select appropriate chemicals according to insect pests. Some chemicals having longer residual action on later growth stages like prothiophos, cartap and fenvalerate mixtures are suitable for management of diamondback moth [19]. Organophosphates (OPs) have been considered as the most important group of compounds for the control of DBM. In OP groups, enough variations in chemical structures have contributed to the wide spectrum of efficacy and varied levels of resistance observed in DBM [20].

5.1. Pyrethoids

Many synthetic pyrethoids (permethrin constituting 0.01%, decamethrin of 0.004%, fenvalerate of 0.01% and cypermethrin of 0.005%) have no good results for controlling after 48 h of the treatment on adult diamondback moth while quinalphos constituting 0.05%, phosalone of 0.05%, endosulfan of 0.05%, monocrotophos of 0.05% and dichlovos of 0.05% have greater toxic effects on both adult and larval stages; after 6 h dichlovos and quinalphos recorded 100% mortality, endosulfan 93% and monocrotophos 63% [21]. Spinosad and permethrins caused 100% mortalities to diamondback moth adults and larvae in leaf dip and residual bioassays method after 72 h of treatment [22].

5.2. Organophosphates

Spinosad and fenvalerate provide good results for the control of diamondback moth larvae at various development stages. Novalurin at 6–12 oz./acre is effective for the control of DBM as compared to non-treated plants, and spinosad is superior to all other insecticides for controlling DBM [23]. Emamectin benzoate with trademark PROCLAIM^{R} is extensively used in the USA and has great degradation on leaf surface and provides good control of DBM larvae and other pest species [24]. Benzoyl phenyl urea and chitin synthesis inhibitors also show good results for controlling resistance-developed population of diamondback moth [25, 26].

5.3. Neem-based insecticides

Neem-based insecticides are most effectively used for the management of *P. xylostella* and other insect pests of Crucifer crops [27, 28]. This type of insecticide, that is, AlignTM (3% formerly agri dyne, Salt Lake City, axadirachtin, Utah), was applied on Lepidopterous pests, mainly *P. xylostella* and other Crucifers crop pests in Texas by [27]. They get results that this insecticide significantly decreases the attack of *P. xylostella* and other insect pests of cabbages and Crucifer crops. Three plant extracts, Annona muricata seeds, *Annona saquamosa* seeds and *Stemona collinsae* roots, are also used at 20 mg/ml concentration and showed high toxic effects, that is, 100% mortality of larvae [29]. The ethyl acetate extracted from *Phytolacca americama* root and extract of Pseudolarix kaempferi, that is, petroleum, is used for the control of DBM larvae; acetate shows stronger insecticidal effects on the second and third instar larvae of *P. xylostella* having LC_{50} values of 225 and 335 ppm [30].

http://dx.doi.org/10.5772/intechopen.74837

6. Biological control of DBM

There are many biological control agents used for the control of diamondback moth including parasitoids and bio-pesticides [31]. In 1998, the main focus was on introducing the two important species of parasitoids, that is, *Diadegma semiclausum* (Ds) and *Diadromus collaris* (Dc), which were introduced from Malaysia by programme for private sector development (PPSD) with the help of FAO Regional Vegetable IPM and CAB International. The parasitoids are successfully established in high-land areas in Vietnam. In particular areas, the lake of effectiveness of parasite or predator control is due to the ability of diamondback moth to migrate and is also established in new planted vegetable areas, and the second important reason for the failure of biological control is the use of highly toxic pesticides in large amounts [32].

Mixture of some chemical and Bt products is very useful for the control of diamondback moth. There is belief that such mixtures are also useful and have large potential for the control of Crucifer insect pests. Similar results was reported as mention above by the use of mixture of typically 20 chemicals formulations [33]. The mixture of Bt products and parasitoids *Diadegma semiclausum* (Ds) and *Diadromus collaris* (Dc) provides effective control of *Plutella xylostella* and other Crucifers crops; the control ranges from 50 to 85% [34]. These mixtures decrease the use of insecticides by 80% in dry season and 55% during rainy season [33]. Mostly, farmers used *Bt* when the attack of DBM larvae exceeded 10/m^2 of crop; farmers used six or seven applications during dry conditions and three or four applications during rainy conditions [35].

6.1. Egg parasitoids

Trichogrammatoidea bactrae is the egg parasitoid of diamondback present naturally in Thailand. This parasite was reared and mass released in the field in mid-1880s and 1990s by the Department of Agriculture, Thailand, and the range of parasitism in unsprayed experimental field is 16–45% of diamondback moth eggs; results show that this parasite controlled DBM but was killed due to chemical spray [36].

6.2. Larval parasitoids

Cotesia plutellae is the larval parasitoid used for the control of diamondback moth (DBM). *Plutella xylostella* L. released without applying insecticides in the glass house has a great effect on the larval stage in Taiwan [37]. In tropical and subtropical areas, where the temperature is greater than 35°C and cauliflower and cabbage are grown, the parasitism of *C. Plutella* was less than 30% [38].

6.3. Pupal parasitoids

Diadromus collaris is the pupal parasite having 6–7 mm of size and only deposits their eggs in the pupa cocoon, having a life cycle of 15 days. This species naturally occurs in Thailand in the province of Chiang Mai and Petchaboon. The parasitism on the pupa of diamondback was studied at the University of Maejo that is 9–30%. Many species like this was observed in February and March in 1990 in Maejo University [36].

7. Bacterial control of DBM

Bacillus thuringiensis as a biopesticide is very good practice to reduce the pest population pressure to cultivate the cruciferous vegetables in cool seasons of many tropical regions [39, 40]. The advantage of *Bt* toxin is that it is extremely precise to its target host especially to DBM. Dry flowable (DF) formulations of Dipel are most compatible with many other insecticides and fungicides. This product is also harmless to the bio-control agents, which are available commercially [41]. Development of resistance in insects is a serious problem against various viruses and *Bt* biopesticide [42]. In many cases, resistance has been observed by DBM against *Bt* toxins. Transgenic Crucifer plants can be used to improve the strategies of resistance management which are applicable broadly to other crops and insects [42]. Three regions of Florida used genetically improved strains of *Bt* and have obtained good results for controlling diamondback moth [43].

8. Nematodial control of diamondback moth

Entomopathogenic nematodes in families Steinernematidae and Heterorhabditidae have great effects for controlling the Lepidopteran pest and the best alternative control by insecticides [44]. It is reported that Steinernematidae, *Steinernema carpocapsae*, is used for the control of diamondback moth [45, 46]. Cell of *X. nematophila* that is present in *S. carpocapsae* is used for the control of diamondback moth larvae [47, 48]. Cell-free solution that contains bacterial cell suspension or nematodes toxins has the best ability for control of diamondback moth larvae [49].

9. Viral control of diamondback moth

Granulosis virus (PxGV), *Autographa californica* nuclear polyhedrosis virus (AcMNPV) and nuclear polyhedrosis virus (GmMNPV) are used for the control of diamondback moth and other cruciferous family crops in Malaysia [50]. Many baculoviruses have been reported for the control of diamondback moth; Granulosis virus (GV) is used for the control of *Plutella xylostella* [51].

10. Resistance against different control strategies

One of the major reasons for the development of resistance to insecticides by DBM is the increasing of number of sprays and thereby increasing cultivation costs. Eco-friendly and less-toxic new chemicals are also available in the market but the farmers are still using broad-spectrum pyrethroids, organophosphates, organochlorines and many other conventional insecticides diamondback moth has developed resistance against these insecticides [52]. Thiodicarb, fipronil, lufenuron, spinosad, carbosulfan and indoxicarb are still performing well as compared to malathion [53]. In Malaysia, high uses of abamectin in Crucifer crops against diamondback moth develop serious problems of resistance [14].

High rate of resistance developed in many insecticides such as cypermethrin, pyrethroids, fenvalerate, organophosphate, deltamethrin and quinalphos was found in DBM population, collected from areas where farmer used mostly pyrethroids at heavy doses [54]. Diamondback moth has developed resistance against fenvalerate, cypermethrin and deltamethrin in the Indian province of Punjab [55]. A new chemical cartap hydrochloride is a successful insecticide for controlling resistance population of DBM. A 170-fold resistance to quinalphos developed in DBM [55].

In some part of the world, DBM became most difficult insects to control because of development of resistance due to the use of extensively toxic chemicals [56, 57]. The extensive use of toxic commercial insecticides against DBM in India is the one of the major constrains in the profitable cultivation of cole crops because these chemicals in heavy and toxic doses developed resistance in DBM [58]. Both mechanisms of resistance and baseline susceptibility are necessary for the effective management of location-specific resistance strategies [59, 60].

Resistances developed 144-fold against diamondback moth due to the use of cyperpethrin at Panipat (Haryana) in India [54]. In DBM, resistance persisted longer in Taiwan against pyrethroids [61]. It is reported that *P. xylostella* is the only pest that develops resistance in the field. OP resistance is not fully investigated and appears probably additional to metabolic resistance mechanisms [62, 63]. The insect growth regulator (IGR) resistance observed in Taiwan DBM populations is significantly affected by piperonyl butoxide action. The synergistic ratios were 7.9:10.4 in three DBM populations for teflubenzuron [64].

The larvae of South Texas strain were less susceptible to indoxacarb than that of the Minnesota strain, and mortality increased with the time of exposure [65]. It is reported that there is no significant difference in the laboratory strain and field population when comparing the resistance [66]. Outside Southeast Asia, it has been reported that there is great development of resistance in this insect pest in several countries, for example, Japan, the USA, Honduras and Australia [67]. In some regions it has been also detected that DBM developed resistance against IGRs which are so-called benzoylphenyl urea (BPUs) [68].

It is documented that difference between two populations of DBM at LC_{50} was 2.9 fold and high levels of resistance developed in DBM against lambda-cyhalothrin and lufenuron [69]. In China, LC_{50} of 1.22, 0.61 and 0.004 ppm against emamectin benzoate from His-Hu strain and Lu-Chu strain and susceptible strain [70].

Author details

Muhammad Imran

Address all correspondence to: imran.bees@gmail.com

Department of Entomology, The University of Poonch, Rawalakot, Azad Jammu and Kashmir, Pakistan

References

[1] Mohan M, Guja GT. Local variation in susceptibility of diamond back moth to insecticides and role of detoxification enzymes. Journal of Crop Protection. 2003;**22**:495-504

[2] Capinera JL. Handbook of Vegetable Pests. Academic Press, San Diego; 2001. 729 p

[3] Huang JW. Advance of studies on insecticide resistance to diamondback moth (*Plutella xylostella* L.). Journal of Guizhou University. 2003;**20**:97-104

[4] Avrdc. Progress Report. Shanhua, Taiwan: Asian Vegetable Research and Development Center; 1987. 480 p

[5] Gujar GT. Farmers fight against diamondback moth (*Plutella xylostella* L.). Pesticides World; 1999. pp. 64-65

[6] Danthanarayana W. Lunar periodicity of insect flight and migration. In: Danthanarayana W, editor. Insect Flight, Dispersal and Migration. Berlin: Springer; 1986. pp. 88-119

[7] Sakanoshita A, Yanagita Y. Fundamental studies on the reproduction of diamondback moth, *Plutella maculipennis* Curtis. I. Effect of environmentla factors on emergence, copulation and oviposition. Proceedings of the Association for Plant Protection of Kyushu. 1985;**18**:11-12

[8] Pivnick KA, Jarvis BJ, Gillott C, Slater GP, Underhill EW. Daily patterns of reproductive activity and the influence of adult density and exposure to host plants on reproduction in the diamondback moth (Lepidoptera: Plutellidae). Environmental Entomology. 1990;**19**: 587-593

[9] Sears MK, Shelton AM. 1985. Evaluation of partial plant sampling procedures and corresponding action thresholds for management of Lepidoptera on cabbage. Journal of Economic Entomology. 1985;**78**:13-16

[10] Harcourt DG. The biology and ecology of the diamondback moth *Plutella xylostella* Curtis, in Eastern Ontario [PhD thesis]. Ithaca, NY: Cornell University; 1954. 107 p

[11] Harcourt DG. Population dynamics of the diamondback moth in Southern Ontario. Diamondback moth management; 1986. pp. 3-15

[12] Kfir R. Origin of the diamondback moth (Lepidoptera: Plutellidae). Annals of the Entomological Society of America. 1998;**91**:164-167

[13] Talekar NS, Shelton AM. Biology, ecology and management of the diamondback moth. Annual Review of Entomology. 1993;**38**:275-301

[14] Verkerk RHJ, Wright DJ. Multi-tropic interactions and management of the diamondback moth: A review. Bulletin of Entomological Research. 1996;**86**:205-216

[15] Walden K. Diamondback Moth (DBM) in Canola. Crop Updates. Western Australia: Department of Agriculture; 2002. pp. 73-78

[16] Talekar NS. Biological control of diamondback moth in Taiwan: A review. Plant Protection Bulletin. 1996;**38**:167-189

[17] Robert HJU, Wright DJ. Multitrophic interactions and management of the diamondback moth a review. Bulletin of Entomological Research. 1996;**86**:205-216

[18] Endersby NM, Ridland PM, Zhang J. Reduced susceptibility to permethrin in diamondback moth populations from vegetable and non-vegetable hosts in Southern Australia. Urania. 2003;**19**:191-201

[19] Nakagome T, Kato K. Control of insects in cruciferous vegetables in Aichi Prefecture with special reference to diamondback moth (In Japanese). In: Insects in Cruciferous Vegetables and their Control with Special Reference to Diamondback Moth. Tokyo: Takeda Chemical Industries Ltd.; 1981. pp. 79-92

[20] Liu MY, Tzeng YJ, Sun CN. Insecticide resistance in the diamondback moth. Journal of Economic Entomology. 1982;**75**:153-155

[21] Mani M, Krishnamoorthy A. Toxicity of some synthetic Pyrethoids and conventional chemical insecticides to the diamondback moth parasite. *Apanteles plutellae* Kurdj. Tropical Pest Management. 1984;**30**:130-132

[22] Travis AH, Foster RE. Effect of insecticides on the diamondback moth and its parasitoid Diadegma insulare (Hymenoptera: Ichneumonidae). Journal of Economic Entomology. 2000;**93**(3):763-768

[23] Dakshina RS. Management of diamondback moth *Plutella xylostella* (L.) (Lepidoptera: Plutellidae) using various chemical practices. Proceedings of the Florida State Horticultural Society. 2003;**116**:54-57

[24] Ronald FL, Dunbar MDM, Minuto LG, Shimabuku RS. Management of diamondback moth with Emamectin benzoate and *Bacillus thuringiensis* subsp. aizawai insecticides. The management of diamondback moth and other crucifer pests; 1997. pp. 178-183

[25] Jansson RK, Lecrone SH. Potential of teflubenzuron for diamondback moth (Lepidoptera: Plutellidae) management on cabbage in Southern Florida. Florida Entomologist. 1988;**71**: 605-615

[26] Perng FS, Sun CN. Susceptibility of diamondback moth (LEPIDOPTERA: PLUTELLIDAE) resistance to conventional insecticide to chitin synthesis inhibitors. Journal of Economic Entomology. 1987;**80**:29-31

[27] Leskovar DI, Boales AK. Azadirachtin potential use for controlling lepidopterous insects and increasing marketability of cabbage. Horticulture Science. 1996;**31**:405-409

[28] Perera DR, Armstrong G, Senanayake N. Effect of antifeedants on the diamondback moth (*Plutellae xylostella*) and its parasitoid *Cotesia plutellae*. Pest Management Science. 2000;**56**: 486-490

[29] Neungpanich S, Roongsook D, Chungsamarnyart N. Insecticidal activity of plant crude extracts on diamondback moth larvae. Witthayasan Kasetsart sakha Witthayasat. 1991;**25**: 106-110

[30] Patcharaporn V, Ding W, Cen XX. Insecticidal activity of five Chinese medicinal plants against *Plutella xylostella* larvae. Journal of Asia-Pacific Entomology. 2010;**13**:169-173

[31] Guan Soon L. Consultancy Report of 4th Mission to The Socialist Republic of Vietnam Agricultural Rehabilitation Project, Plant Protection Sub-Component: Integrated Pest Management in Vegetables. IIBC Malaysia Regional Station: CAB International; 1997. 31 p

[32] Bretherton RF. Lepidoptera immigration to the British isles, 1969 to 1977. Proceedings and Transactions of the British Entomological and Natural History Society. 1982;**15**:98-110

[33] Huong LTT. Integrated pest management in cabbage: Guiding documents of agro-ecosystems on growing, developing, practice methods, pest management and diseases, pests, natural enemies in cabbage. IPM-FAO Vegetables Program in South and Southeast; 2004. 113 p

[34] Nga LT. The role of biological control in crucifer production: A case study of *Bacillus thuringiensis* usage in crucifer pest management of diamondback moth in the city area, Lam Dong Province, Vietnam [MSc thesis]. Asian Institute of Technology. AS-06-12. 2006. 108 p

[35] Attique MNR, Khaliq A, Sayyed AH. Could resistance to insecticides in *Plutella xylostella* (Lep., Plutellidae) be overcome by insecticide mixtures. Journal of Applied Entomology. 2006;**130**:122-127

[36] Brent R. Parasitoids of the DBM in Thailand Dept. of Horticulture, University of Kentucky. 2004. Available from: http://thailand.ipm/natural_enemies /DBM_parasitoids.htm

[37] Min K, Seung H, Mei-Ying L. An evidence to use *Cotesia plutellae* (Kurdjumov) (Hymenoptera: Braconidae) as a field control agent against diamondback moth, *Plutella xylostella* L. (Lepidoptera: Plutellidae). Journal of Asia-Pacific Entomology. 2006;**9**(1):55-59

[38] Waladde SM, Leutle MF, Villet MH. Parasitism of diamondback moth, *Plutella xylostella* L. (Lepidoptera: Yponomeutidae); field and laboratory observations. Journal of African Tydskr Plant Ground. 2001;**18**:32-37

[39] Amend J, Basedow TH. Combining release/establishment of *Diadegma semiclausum* (Helle'n) (HymL: Ichneumonidae) and *Bacillus thuringiensis* Berl. for control of *Plutella xylostella* (L.) (Lep: Yponomeutidae) and other lepidopteron pests in the Cordillera region of Luzon (Philippines). Journal of Applied Entomology. 1997;**121**:337-342

[40] Saucke H, Dori F, Schmutterer H. Biological and integrated control of *Plutella xylostella* (Lep: Yponomeutidae) and Crocidolomia pavonana (Lep: Pyralidae) in *Brassica* crops in Papua New Guinea. Biocontrol Science and Technology. 2000;**10**:595-606

[41] Singh SP, Jalali SK, Venkatesan T. Susceptibility of diamondback moth and its egg parasitoid to a new Bt formulation. Journal of Pest Management in Horticultural Ecosystems. 2000;**6**(2):114-116

[42] Shelton A. Potential of *Bt Brassica* Vegetables, Project Done with an Indian university. 2004. Available from: http://www.nysaes.cornell.edu/ent/faculty/abstract.html

[43] Leibee GL, Jansson RR, Foster RE, Daoust RA. Evaluation of new *Bacillus thuringiensis* based insecticides for control of lepidopterous pests of cabbage in Florida. Florida Entomologist. 1990;**85**:215-219

[44] Kaya HK, Gaugler R. Entomopathogenic nematodes. Annual Review of Entomology. 1993;**38**:181-206

[45] Morris ON. Susceptibility of 31 species of agricultural insect pests to entomopathogenic nematodes Steinernema feltiae and *Heterorhabditis bacteriophora*. The Canadian Entomologist. 1985;**117**:401-407

[46] Ratnasinghe G, Hague, NGM. Efficacy of entomopathogenic nematodes against the diamondback moth, Plutella xylostella (Lepidoptera: Yponomeutidae). Pakistan Journal of Nematology. 1997;**15**:45-53

[47] Boemare NE, Givaudan A, Brehelin M, Laumond C. Symbiosis and pathogencity of nematode bacterium complexes. Symbiosis. 1997;**22**:21-45

[48] Elawad SA. Studies on the taxonomy and biology of a newly isolated species of Steinernema (Steinernematidae: Nematoda) from the tropics and its associated bacteria [PhD thesis]. Department of Agriculture, University of Reading, UK. 1998

[49] Mahar AN, Munir M, Sami E, Nigel H. Microbial control of diamondback moth, *Plutella xylostella* L. (Lepidoptera: Yponomeutidae) using bacteria (*Xenorhabdus nematophila*) and its metabolites from the entomopathogenic nematode *Steinernema carpocapsae*. Journal of Zhejiang University-SCIENCE. 2004;**5**(10):1183-1190

[50] Hussan AK. Potential of several Baculoviruses for the control of diamondback moth and Crocidolomia binotalis on cabbages basic research division, MARDI, Serdang. Journal of Applied Entomology. 2001;**86**:20-24

[51] Asayama T, Osaki N. A granulosis virus of the diamondback moth, *Plutella xylostella* (L.) (maculipennis Curt.) (Plutellidae: Lepidoptera). Research Bulletin Aichi Ken Agriculture Research Center. 1969;**1**:45-54

[52] Kumara AVK. Externalities in the use of pesticides: An economic analysis in a cole crop [MSc (Agri.) thesis]. (Unpublished), U.A.S. Bangalore, India. 1995

[53] Vastrad AS, Lingappa S, Basavanagoud K. Management of insecticide resistant populations of diamondback moth. Journal of Pest Management and Horticulture Ecosystem. 2003;**1**:33-40

[54] Saxena JD, Rai S, Srivastava KM, Sinha SR. Resistance in the field population of the diamondback moth to some commonly used synthetic pyrethroids. Indian Journal of Entomology. 1989;**51**(265):268

[55] Joia BS, Udeaan AS, Chawla RP. Laboratory evaluation of cartap hydrochloride an alternative promising insecticide against multi-resistant populations of diamondback moth in Punjab. In: Natl. Symp. On Emerging Trends in Pest Management, Solan. 1994. pp. 28-30

[56] Shelton AM, Sances FV. Assessment of insecticide resistance after the outbreak of diamondback moth (Lepidoptera: Plutellidae) in California. Journal of Economic Entomology. 2000;**93**:931-936

[57] Sarfraz M, Keddie BA. Conserving the efficacy of insecticides against *Plutella xylostella* (L) (Lepidoptera Plutellidae). Journal of Applied Entomology. 2005;**129**:49-157

[58] Georghiou GP. Overview of insecticide. In: Managing Resistance in Agro-Chemical from Fundamental Research to Practical Strategies. Washington DC: Amercian Society; 1990. pp. 18-41

[59] Denholm I, Rowland MW. Tactics for managing pesticide resistance in arthropods: Theory and practice. Annual Review of Entomology. 1992;**37**:91-112

[60] Denholm I, Pickett JA, Devonshire AL. Insecticide Resistance: From Mechanisms to Management. London: CAB International and Royal Society; 1999. 123 p

[61] Chen CN, Sun WY. Ecology and control threshold of the diamondback moth on crucifers in Taiwan, in diamondback moth management. In: Talekar NS, Griggs TG, editors. Proceedings of the 1st International Workshop Taiwan, Asian Vegetable Research and Development Center. Mar 11–15, 1986

[62] Sayyed AH, Ferre J, Wright DJ. Mode of inheritance and stability of resistance to *Bacillus thuringiensis* var. kurstaki in a diamondback moth (*Plutella xylostella*) population from Malaysia. Pest Management Science. 2000;**56**:743-748

[63] Sayyed AH, Harward R, Herrero S, Ferre J, Wright DJ. Genetic and biochemical approach for characterization of resistance to *Bacillus thuringiensis* toxin CrylAc is a field population of the diamondback moth. Applied and Environmental Microbiology. 2000;**66**:1509-1516

[64] Cheng EY, Kao CH, Chiu CS. Insecticide resistance study in *Plutella xylostella* L. the IGR-resistance and the possible management strategy. Journal of Agricultural Research of China. 1990;**39**:208-220

[65] Liu TX, Hutchison WD, Chen W, Burkness EC. Comparative susceptibilities of diamondback moth (Lepidoptera: Plutella) and cabbage looper (Lepidopter: Noctuidae) from Minnesota and South Texas to λ-cyhalothrin and indoxacarb. Journal of Economic Entomology. 2003;**94**(4):1230-1236

[66] Shelton AM, Robertson JL, Tang JD, Perez C, Eigenbrode SD, Preisler HK, Wilsey WT, Cooley RJ. Resistance of diamondback moth (Lepidoptera: Plutellidae) to *Bacillus thuringiensis* subspecies in the field. Journal of Economic Entomology. 1993;**86**:697-705

[67] Secaira E. Panamerican College of Agriculture, Zamorano, Honduras. Personal Communication. 1988

[68] Lin JG, Hung CF, Sun CN. Teflubenzuron resistance and microsomal monooxygenases in larvae of the diamondback moth. Pesticide Biochemistry and Physiology. 1989;**35**:20-25

[69] Cho YS, Lee SC. Resistance development and cross resistance of diamondback moth *Plutella xylostella* (Lepidoptera: Plutellidae) by the application of single selection for several insecticides. Korean Journal of Applied Entomology. 1994;**33**:242-249

[70] Löhr B, Gathu R, Kariuki C, Obiero J, Gichini G. Impact of an exotic parasitoid on *Plutella xylostella* (Lepidoptera: Plutellidae) population dynamics, damage and indigenous natural enemies in Kenya. Bulletin of Entomological Research. 2007;**97**:337-350